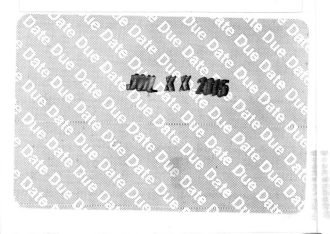

Women
Living with
Self-Injury

Women
Living with
Self-Injury

Jane Wegscheider Hyman

Temple University Press   *Philadelphia*

Temple University Press, Philadelphia 19122
Copyright © 1999 by Jane Wegscheider Hyman
All rights reserved
Published 1999
Printed in the United States of America

⊗ The paper used in this publication meets the requirements of
American National Standard for Information Sciences — Permanence
of Paper for Printed Library Materials, ANSI Z39.48-1984

Library of Congress Cataloging-in-Publication Data

Hyman, Jane Wegscheider.
    Women living with self-injury / Jane Wegscheider Hyman.
        p. cm.
    ISBN 1-56639-720-0 (cloth : alk. paper). — ISBN 1-56639-721-9 (pbk. : alk. paper)
    1. Self-mutilation.   2. Women — Mental health.   3. Self-injurious behavior.
I. Title.
    RC552.S4H95   1999
    616.85′82′0082 — dc21   99-17714
                                                                          CIP

If you could come into my mind and see what I see—
I'm trying to let you see what I see.

Elizabeth

This book is dedicated to the women
whose experiences made it possible,

and, as always, to
JFH and HW.

Wer die Fragen nicht beantworten kann,

hat die Pruefung bestanden.

Franz Kafka, *Die Pruefung*, 1936

Contents

Acknowledgments

THIS PROJECT was possible because of my informants: the women who taught me what it is like to live with and overcome self-injury. My first thanks go to them for their honesty, courage, patience, and trust, and for allowing me to be their scribe. Several of them became my editors as well, critiquing the chapters they helped create and patiently allowing me to call them again and again, long after the original interviews, to check on uncertainties. They also became role models because of their fortitude and lack of self-pity. I regret that they cannot be thanked by name.

As always, Mary Waggener, Charles Hyman, Jack Hyman, Peggy Schoditsch, and Sonja Wetzsteon provided interest, encouragement, and sensitive chapter critiques. Andee Rubin, long-time friend and "personal editor," allowed me once again to benefit from her skill in chapter structure and organization, and to enjoy her empathic interest. My special thanks also to Sarah Shaw, Susan Lewis, and Barent Walsh with whom I meet monthly to discuss aspects of self-injury and our respective work on the subject. We provide each other with challenges, disagreements, endless questions, critiques of chapter and article drafts, and opportunities to talk about self-injury, not a topic our friends or colleagues necessarily want to discuss. Susan and Barent critiqued several chapters each, and Sarah critiqued drafts of all chapters. Dawn Balcazar and Robin Connors took the time to review the book proposal as well as critique later chapters, and Dawn Balcazar reviewed the entire first draft. Ruta Mazelis gave her valuable critique to the first four chapters. Of course, my gratitude to all those mentioned above and below does not imply that they agree with me on all points, or that errors are anyone's fault but my own.

Michael Ames, my editor, amazed me during our first conversation because our views on why this type of book should be written coincided exactly. I had never heard such an empathic response from an editor, and I chose Temple University Press largely because of Michael. Throughout this project he was insightful and objective, yet showed his essential trust in my judgment, goals, and work methods, for which I am grateful.

Parts of this project date back to my dissertation years of the early to mid 1990s—a late-life dissertation—and to the valuable critical readings of the dissertation committee members Penny MacElveen-Hoehn, Ross V. Speck, Emily Fox Kales, Judith Sanditen, Judith Beth Cohen, and Demetria Iazetto. The origins of the project are even earlier, when Jan Brin, an advocate for self-injuring women, first introduced me to the subject and insisted that self-injury deserves public attention. Jan eventually put me in touch with self-injuring women for interviews, critiqued several chapters, and gave me the idea of including chapters written entirely in women's own voices. Later disagreements ended our communications, and Jan may not share many of the views expressed in this book, which nonetheless owes so much to her.

Others who donated their time and expertise by critiquing chapter drafts are Caroline Caswell, Judith Beth Cohen, Michael de Bellis, William Kadish, Deb Martinson, Dennis McCrory, Bradford D. Reich, Kristy Trautmann, and Iris Weaver. Additional people sent studies and gave generously of their time and expertise by phone. My thanks to you all.

Introduction

. . . .

Elizabeth: When I first started hurting myself, I was a teenager and I did it using hammers. If there was a scene in the house with my dad—because he was violent—I would go upstairs and I would be so frustrated, but it seemed like it was *stuck* here in my chest. And I would bang my head against a wall, or get his hammer from the toolshed and beat on myself. It didn't feel weird, and after I did it, I didn't say: "Oh my God! What the heck am I doing? This is not right." Because it felt good, and it helped me vent my frustration and my anger. And it kind of became a habit then. But it never seemed like it was out of the ordinary because I never told anybody up until two years ago. No one in the entire universe knew before that. It was just my thing, so there was nobody to tell me that it was weird. And it felt good to me, so I wasn't going to say it was weird. It was only when people found out about it and were saying that that was extreme behavior and it's called "self-destructiveness" and "self-injury" and all these *labels.* Then I realized it was wrong, but even then, I was like: "I don't care. It feels good."

. . . .

ELIZABETH IS one of fifteen women whose experiences of living with self-injury shaped this book. Like countless others, these women cut their arms and legs with knives and razors; scratch at their skin; burn, bruise, or stick themselves with cigarettes, hammers, pins, and other objects; bang their heads and limbs; and break their own bones. Concealing any resulting scars or other signs of injury is crucial and partly dictates their daily routines, choice of clothes, and choice of an appropriate lie to excuse any traces of injury that have to remain visible. When I spoke with them, the majority had already been living with self-injury for thirteen years or longer while simultaneously working outside the home and, in some cases, raising children. Throughout this book they speak, secure in their anonymity from a public that generally sees self-injury as frightening, senseless, and repulsive.

Most of these women have lived with self-injury during their years of greatest sexual and professional potential, making self-injury a possible force in their working lives and in their relationships with partners, children, and friends. All fifteen women work outside the home; six had sexual partners at the time of the interview, and six are mothers. One chapter is devoted to self-injuring women at the workplace and another to the effects of self-injury on women's personal relationships.

1

I found these women eager for a book that would explain the logic of their "weird" actions, give dignity to their behavior, and discuss their concerns as workers, partners, friends, and mothers. Because I am an independent researcher interested in the ways self-injury affects the quality of women's lives, I asked questions they had never been asked before. One woman said that she told me more than she had ever told her therapist. Because I am a writer specializing in women's health, these women hoped that their experiences would reach the public and increase awareness and understanding of self-injury. Because I am a woman who lived with obsessive-compulsive disorder half of her life, some of the women I interviewed may have sensed that I could listen and understand without judging.

Through an acquaintance who used to injure herself, word of mouth, advertisements in a women's newspaper, and posted fliers, I found and interviewed twenty women ages twenty-five to fifty-one, all living in the northeast or on the west coast of the United States at the time of the interviews. Fifteen of these women's stories constitute the bulk of the text. Supplementary information stems from professional journal articles and from women who formerly or currently self-injure and are now advocates for other women who injure themselves.

Through years of writing on women's health I was experienced in asking potentially embarrassing questions about topics women rarely discuss. Yet, finding women willing to confide in me was not simple. I had underestimated the level of shame attached to self-injury and the fear women had of repelling me by graphic descriptions of their diverse methods of injuring themselves. For some women, scheduling the actual interview was a major and somewhat frightening step. Talking openly about the subject was an experience some had never had except with their therapists or, perhaps, with other women who self-injure. Some were visibly moved while telling what they do to themselves and about their childhood experiences. In the middle of the interview one woman said, "I can't believe I'm telling you these things."

I conducted the interviews during meetings or by telephone, with each interview taking around three hours. The interview consisted of audio-taped, open-ended questions that I had constructed over a period of months based on prior years of reading on self-injury and on a pilot study. The audiotapes were then transcribed into text, which I analyzed for themes and patterns and from which this book is compiled. I tried to capture the women's own powerful words as much as possible, either directly or by paraphrasing: three chapters are entirely in the women's own words from interviews that I edited and rearranged in narrative form; direct quotes make up large parts of most other chapters. Each woman also filled out a brief questionnaire on personal and family background and on therapies for self-injury. When I began the writing process, women who were still reachable and willing critiqued at least one chapter-draft each, providing valuable additions and corrections.

During my original search for informants, I looked for women who work outside the home and who had been repeatedly cutting, hitting, burning, or otherwise injuring themselves for at least one year. Later in the process I included women who had stopped so that they could tell about the methods they use to keep themselves free of self-injury. No other limitations were set but the study is, nonetheless, circumscribed. With one exception, every woman who responded had experienced prolonged sexual, physical, or emotional abuse as a child. For the first few years of my research, I believed there was an almost inevitable connection between self-injury and prior abuse. This is not the case. Repeated childhood illnesses or hospitalizations, chronic family chaos, separations from a caregiver, and witnessing violence can all lead to self-injury. Demeaning experiences concerning an adolescent girl's changing body — such as comments, insinuations, insults, or unwanted exposure — may also result in self-injury, especially if a girl feels that she cannot use words to convey the distress such intrusions cause her. For some girls, self-injury may become a general form of self-expression when they doubt or do not recognize their own feelings and experiences.[1] A girl who does not cut or burn herself may be friends with one who does and begin self-injuring by copying her friend's methods of coping in times of stress. This may be one reason self-injury appears to be spreading. Sometimes self-injury among adolescent girls disappears when they enter their late teens or early twenties. Nonetheless, prolonged childhood physical, sexual, or emotional abuse or neglect precedes self-injury for many, perhaps most, women who live with self-injury in adulthood, such as the women who entrusted their experiences to me. The prologue and chapter two illustrate the many links between childhood abuse and self-injury.

All women who responded to my search were Caucasian Americans of European descent. Women of non-European origin also injure themselves, yet they appear in studies either in very small numbers or not at all, and no one knows if they are equally prone to injuring themselves.[2] Their scarcity in research could reflect a tendency to express emotional distress in other ways, but it could also reflect a reluctance to participate in studies or to seek help from psychiatric hospitals primarily run by European Americans. Because of these limitations in ethnicity and childhood experiences, this book reflects self-injury in the lives of formerly abused, active, adult women of European origin, women in whose lives self-injury has been a central but hidden factor for years. Men are excluded because self-injury appears to be primarily a woman's coping strategy, at least among those who seek help from therapists.[3] Some of the possible reasons for a gender split are discussed in chapter two.

When I was well into the analysis of the transcribed interviews, a woman called me in response to a flier she had seen about my study. She told me that she compulsively squeezed the skin of her breasts. Yet, the reasons she gave for doing this and what she felt afterward did not correspond with the information from the nineteen women I had already interviewed. This woman's experiences made me struggle again with a definition for self-injury.

How to define self-injury remains one of the many unanswered questions about it. Psychologists and psychiatrists tend to define actions such as self-cutting, -hitting, and -burning as deliberate, repetitive, and socially unacceptable harm to one's body without a conscious intent to die,[4] a definition I use for lack of a better one. Yet, there are countless actions that could be defined in such a way. Pulling out one's hair is sometimes considered a form of self-injury, but I agree with others who see it as a different, though sometimes overlapping, problem called trichotillomania. Actions such as compulsively squeezing the skin to the point of leaving scars or biting nails until the fingers bleed are sometimes associated with trichotillomania but could also be called self-injury. Drinking alcoholic beverages mixed with shampoo, super glue, brake fluid, insecticide, or "anything that burns" could be called self-injury, alcoholism, or both.[5] Depriving oneself of food or gorging on it and then vomiting or taking laxatives could be called anorexia and bulimia respectively, self-injury, or both.

The provision of mental health services in the United States is often based on the belief that thoughts and actions can be accurately defined. Giving acts such as self-cutting, -hitting, and -burning a name is useful mainly for therapists, who rely on the theory that proper diagnostic categories lead to proper therapy, and for medical insurance employees, who require diagnostic categories to reimburse the cost of professional intervention. Over the years, mental health practitioners have tried to categorize and define self-cutting, -hitting, -burning, or otherwise injuring the body by relating these actions to schizophrenia, psychosis, or neurosis. Currently, therapists commonly classify self-injury as a sign of borderline personality disorder and a disorder of impulse control "not otherwise specified," but also as associated with posttraumatic stress disorder.[6] Similarly, mental health practitioners have given such actions an array of names: self-mutilation, autoaggression, symbolic wounding, self-attack, self-inflicted violence, self-abuse, focal suicide, attempted suicide, suicidation, parasuicide, antisuicide, wrist-cutting syndrome, wrist slashing, delicate self-cutting syndrome, self-assault, chronic repetitive self-injury, carving, indirect self-destructive behavior, deliberate self-harm, and self-injury.

Yet, the actions themselves have a way of spilling out of diagnostic containers and mixing with each other until they are indistinguishable. For example, some women say that they starve themselves to be thin, are driven to binge-eat because their bodies are starving, then purge to avoid weight gain. Others say that they deny themselves food or purge whatever they do eat to hurt their bodies, or that they eat compulsively or in binges to relieve stress, block out emotional pain, become fat and therefore unattractive to men, or escape a less intense numbness than the numbness they escape through cutting themselves. Some women who pull out their hair do so to assuage emotional pain, but also because they happen to look in the mirror and fall into a trance-like state of constant hair-pulling. Yet, they also pull out their hair when they are relaxed, as though their hands had become independent and could not be still. Women who cut, hit, or burn themselves do so to feel that they are inside their bodies but also to "leave" their bodies, to release emotions, to see blood, to punish themselves, to avoid suicide, to ask for help without using words, to reorganize turbulent thoughts, to make emotional pain concrete, and for other reasons. These and other forms of temporary self-help are strikingly versatile, defying strict categories.

As a researcher, I had to accept this versatility and the impossibility of adequately defining self-injury. I also had to learn the differences between women's own terms for what they do and the terms used within the fields of psychology and psychiatry. At the beginning, I assumed that self-injury was an act with only the negative consequences of secrecy, shame, and mortification. Social ostracism, I thought, could be added to the list of negatives because compulsive actions that leave visible marks on the body are stigmatizing. I became interested in self-injury partly because it is considered socially unacceptable yet can leave telltale traces on the body. From my own experiences with obsessive-compulsive disorder, I knew that a socially unacceptable compulsion is hard enough to bear even when it leaves no visible traces. What must it be like, I wondered, to live with it written on the body? What if friends see the scars and bruises? Do scars affect women's options in getting a job, finding a loving partner, raising children? I conjectured that partly because of its potential visibility, women would want to rid themselves of self-injury if they could.

Though some of my assumptions proved true, I soon learned that self-injury can be necessary and beneficial to the point of saving a woman from suicide, or even from homicide. Erica, one of my informants, chastised me early in our interview sessions for assuming that negative terms such as "deliberate self-harm" and "self-injury," which I had learned from reading professional journals, were appropriate terms to choose from:

. . . .

I'd like to have a little semantic discussion. I recognize that this stuff is perceived as harmful, but I don't see it that way. For the benefit of communication, I will use that terminology, but for me, the benefits outweigh the harms.
And I suppose, to be perfectly truthful, I would like that balance to tip: I
would like the harms to outweigh the benefits so that there was some real
gain to be had by stopping.

. . . .

In this book I use the term "self-injury" because I find it the least offensive
general term already in use and accepted by some women who self-injure. I
regret that this term was not introduced by the women themselves and that it
has solely negative connotations.

None of the labels that I or many others use necessarily reflect how a self-
injuring woman sees her actions. Some self-injuring women perceive from
the beginning that their actions are outside the social norm. Yet to others, self-
injury initially feels like a normal, necessary way of expressing emotions, like
shouting or crying. Gradually, they realize how the actions that seem normal
to them are perceived by others. Thereafter, it is difficult for these self-injuring
women to see their actions as strictly positive acts, although some women say
that public condemnation is still the only negative aspect of self-injury and is
the main reason they want to stop:

. . . .

Edith: When I finally came to realize that this was not quite normal
behavior . . . it was awful for me because I felt so guilty about it, and so
wrong. . . . So, my thought is, I *have* to get rid of this [open wound from
scratching] but where can I have one that no one will see? Which is very
hard to admit because this is crazy: You want to get rid of this one but you
don't want to *stop*, you just want to have one someplace that nobody can
see! . . . Because, still, for me, the only part that I don't like about it is that it's
visible to other people. I suppose there's a small part of me inside that says:
"You know this isn't normal. . . ." I think that the major reason I want to stop
is simply because it's abnormal, and it's weird, and I don't want to have all
these scars.

. . . .

Because self-injury is beneficial in so many ways, some women feel conflicted: while acknowledging that others consider their actions abnormal and
self-destructive, they may partly accept the negative views, yet defend self-

injury as a viable, necessary form of self-help. Here, Elizabeth expresses the pull she feels between social condemnation and her own perceptions of self-injury:

. . . .

I've gotten so used to doing it now, it's like it's a part of me. For me, it seems normal to go up and lock myself in my room, and take out my razor blades, and cut. I don't see that it's abnormal, I don't see that it's crazy, because it's part of me and I've been doing it for so long. I remember starting it when I was fifteen, right after my brother abused me, and I've been doing it ever since. I feel so calm after I do it. People who don't do it, they don't understand that. It's hard to make them understand. . . .

I couldn't see why [my counselor] would call it abnormal. Because she said, "First there's the normal range and then there's crazy." And I said, "Hold on a second! If that's not in the normal range that means it's in the crazy range, and I'm not crazy. I'm completely sane: I hold down a good job, I manage my finances well—a crazy person couldn't do that." So, I know I'm not crazy, and my behavior is not crazy. I don't care what anybody says; I think it's normal. I know that a lot of people would disagree, but I think that other people who do this would agree.

. . . .

Erica is one who agrees. She says that she has always known that self-injury is an irreplaceable benefit in her life. Simultaneously, she has kept it hidden, tacitly admitting that "this is not good." In what way is it not good? Some women who injure themselves point out that smoking cigarettes is considered normal, yet it is far more harmful to the body than cutting, hitting, burning, or picking. Ironically, self-injury involves less harm than many other methods of disguising or releasing emotions. The drama of attacking one's own body, and the blood and scars that can result, are misleading: usually the skin's natural capacity to heal itself takes care of the damage. Even self-inflicted wounds requiring stitches do not usually entail serious, long-term harm to the body, while smoking cigarettes and abusing alcohol do.

Barbara, who has used food, alcohol, and other mind-altering substances to live with unbearable memories and emotions says that cutting is the most direct and least harmful method. It does not harm her liver, like alcohol, or her teeth, stomach, and balance of electrolytes, like vomiting after binge-eating. She admits that she would prefer being addicted to something healthful, such as swimming or riding a bike, but points out that anything that becomes a compulsion is not life-affirming:

. . . .

There are compulsive joggers out there or . . . people who are just doing; compulsive doers. They're not really feeling their feelings and living their lives. They are just acting out in socially acceptable ways. . . . You're not allowing what's there to be there if you have to run out and jog every minute. It just looks better and people don't mind seeing it as much as they mind seeing cutting. They get proud of it. Like you see someone who is anorexic even, and you go, "Oh wow, you're so skinny!" The person is purging or taking laxatives and all these terrible things, but they *look* good. Like the compulsive doers: "Wow, you got so much done!" Meantime, the person can't even deal with their kids or anything else because they are so hung up on do, do, do; they're just trying to avoid their feelings. There are all different ways to do it. . . .

My therapist [once] said: "What would your words be if you weren't just cutting; what would you be saying?" I got out a whole lot of stuff that I wasn't saying because I was cutting. I didn't have to say it because I cut it away. Just like you think you have a drink and your problems go away; well, you never had to deal with them because you drink. Your feelings went away—but it is just temporary.

. . . .

Here, Barbara defends self-injury as one of the least harmful addictions, and also reveals her conflict: self-injury may be relatively healthy, but she would rather be able to tolerate her feelings and express them in words.

Descriptive terms that mental health practitioners use, such as self-mutilation, emphasize harm done to the body. However, the women these professionals are studying have strikingly different descriptive terms for their actions: "friend," "crutch," "security blanket," "life-preserver," "vent," "medication," "validation." All these terms refer to people, objects, substances, or actions that help one get through difficult times. Because women have not been asked for their own terms for what they do, their voices have not been heard; because their actions are secret, their descriptive terms are often not familiar even to each other. Women's positive terms, however, are often followed by terms that express conflict and lack of choice because a woman who injures herself usually feels that she cannot stop. She may also find that self-injury keeps her from learning socially acceptable ways of coping, or that it perpetuates the violence done to her body in the past. It is understandable that Barbara, who calls self-injury a "life-preserver," also calls it her "ball and chain"; and Elizabeth, who calls self-injury a "friend," also calls it a "demon."

Some women express their lack of choice by calling their actions compulsive, and their thoughts obsessive, because self-injury can take over a woman's thoughts against her will. Self-injury is, however, not the same as the anxiety-driven washing, cleaning, or checking characteristic of obsessive-compulsive disorder, although some women have signs of both problems.[7] Women sometimes find that the term "impulse" describes an act of self-injury, especially the quick, unpremeditated actions often involved in picking or hitting. The term "impulse" is, however, inappropriate for those self-injuring actions thought of and planned hours in advance. Some women find that "addiction" best fits the overall experience of self-injury, no matter what the specific action may be. First, many women switch from alcohol or other drug addictions to self-injury, suggesting that self-injury is a substitute drug. Second, for some women, self-injury becomes a way of responding to almost any emotional stress, just as drugs and alcohol seem to do. Possibly, the body becomes dependent on internal painkillers secreted in response to self-injury, just as it can become dependent on the soothing properties of alcohol, nicotine, and other drugs.

Although "addiction" may often be a useful category for self-injury, it too does not comfortably fit all women. Self-injury is as complex and diverse as the women who experience it and seems to defy any single descriptive term. Esther has her own term, the one perhaps most fitting to many women who chronically self-injure.

· · · · · · · · ·

I don't know if I'd call it an addiction, because to me, [with] an addiction . . . you start out using alcohol or drugs to get through a certain thing and then it turns out that you are not just using it for that anymore, you are using it for everything, an all-the-time thing. Whereas I still use cutting, hitting, and pinching for . . . just getting through those tough times. I guess the biggest thing I would call it is — this sounds funny — salvation. Even though I know that it's a "bad" thing to do, it's kept me alive.

· · · · · · · · ·

Esther, Barbara, Elizabeth, and Erica, like all my informants, hope that this book, with their own words and experiences, will promote understanding and compassion for self-injury and help break down secrecy and shame. They want to be able to be truthful about their actions with friends, families, co-workers, physicians, and therapists. As Esther says:

· · · · · · · · ·

Maybe [this book] could teach people the truth about what it is and what it isn't. They get the wrong idea about it and they're horrified. I'd like to see that change because one thing that we don't need is to be pulled away from — like it's a disease somebody's going to catch, or like we're homicidal instead of just injuring ourselves. It would be nice to say "These are scars from my knife or from a razor blade" and have a person not think "Oh, how horrible, how disgusting! How can you do that to *yourself?*"

. . . .

These women's involvement in this book is a way of breaking their own and other self-injuring women's isolation. If the book reaches mental health professionals, physicians, and schoolteachers as well, they, in turn, can help girls and women who injure themselves. Two chapters are devoted to recovery methods, including self-help, and one of those chapters includes self injuring women's advice to therapists. As Edith says: "Maybe we'll put this all together someday and figure out how to help us not just stop it, but stop *needing* to do it." I share these hopes for this book and add one more: that it will encourage awareness of the one to three million U.S. children abused yearly, of which close to one thousand die of the immediate causes of abuse and countless others die of abuse-related suicide.[8] Among those children who managed to stay alive, grow up, and become full participants in society are the women who describe their lives on the following pages.

Interviewees

The ages and professions of my informants at the time of the interviews are as follows, listed in the chronological order of the interviews, using the names they chose or that I chose for them:

Edith, 51, physical therapist

Karen, 49, human services worker

Elizabeth, 25, typist

Jane, 39, treasurer

Erica, 43, editor and writer

Peggy, 34, human services worker

Barbara, 38, social worker

Mary, 47, technology manager for communications company

Esther, 40, central security station operator and store sales associate

Jessica, 46, part-time social worker and in graduate school for social work

Rosa, 30, drafter for engineering and architectural firm
Meredith, 26, part-time social worker and in graduate school for social work
Caroline, 30, office staff worker and student in music school
Helena, 28, freelance proofreader and copyeditor
Sarah O., 27, part-time worker while in graduate school in pharmacy

Prologue

Home, Sweet Home

· · · · · · · · ·

Elizabeth: There's a lot that I can't remember. Sometimes I'll get just one picture of things in my mind and I can't remember the whole incident. I have one picture of me and my younger sister in the bathtub, and my dad touching us. I don't remember how it felt when he was doing it to me, but I remember how it felt when I watched him doing it to my sister. And it felt probably worse, because I knew it was wrong, and I couldn't stop it.

My dad would beat us. He would go into these *rages* where, if we stepped out of line, there would be slaps across the face, punches. He would trap us in a corner and punch us, kick us. I hated my dad, and I still do. When I call home, I don't talk to him. He's not part of my life anymore.

When I was fifteen, my brother raped me. I used to share a room with my sister, and my sister was gone away for the night. I was kind of nervous on my own because I come from a large family, and I had shared a room with some-one all my life. My brother had been out drinking, drugging—which I didn't know. When I heard him come home I was relieved because I felt safe. But I kept hearing noises outside, and I don't know if that was just me being para-noid. He came into my room, and I told him I was scared. He said he'd stay with me for a while—but if he was going to stay with me, he wanted to get under the covers. So I said "Okay."

It's hard, because it's not something one can share with someone. After ev-erything happened, I've never felt like I've been cleansed of it. It's still on me; it's still there. . . . I know that's why I cut. It's almost like I'm trying to cleanse my body of it, trying to get rid of it.

• • •

Edith: When I was very young my father started putting things inside me, sexually stimulating me. It finally grew to rape. I wasn't very old when he penetrated for the first time with his penis—I guess that I was around three or four. And when that memory came back there was this awful cracking sound but there was absolutely no sensation of pain. I've had bladder surgery, because probably there was some damage to my bladder.

If my mother knew that my father was doing anything with me, afterward she'd come back and hit [me]. Probably the most horrible memory of her—

and I don't have that many—was when my father had done oral sex for the first time. I got sick afterwards; I was throwing up. And she came in and was *wild*. . . . She was not normally a screamer or a yeller. Normally, if I did anything that was wrong she'd just withdraw and wouldn't talk to me until I would apologize no matter what it was; whether *she* had done it, *I* had to apologize before she would be available at all for anything. Basically, the less I needed her, the more available she was; and if I really needed her, she wasn't available at all. I learned real quickly not to need her. But that particular time, I was lying on a little rug that was next to my bed, and she came in hitting, kicking, yelling, screaming. That's the only way she knew how to deal with it, I guess. . . . She also used to give me enemas on a general basis when I was a kid. Not several every day, but often enough that it was painful.

· · · · · · · · · ·

LIKE ELIZABETH and Edith, many women who chronically injure themselves were repeatedly abused as children.[1] Often they were abused by the very people they depended on for their welfare and safety and whom they were taught to love and obey: parents, grandparents, stepparents, and older siblings.[2] Their experiences include genital fondling and rape; random physical attacks; physical neglect, abuse, and torture; physical and sexual abuse within the context of rituals; and emotional abuse and neglect.

Chronic abuses within families are among the most severe traumas that we can experience.[3] Women are more likely than men to experience sexual abuse, both as children and as adults. Although boys and girls suffer almost equally from physical abuse, girls are two to three times more likely to be sexually abused,[4] and far more girls than boys are victims of incest. Childhood abuse is also associated with subsequent depression, anxiety, volatile emotions, dissociation, eating problems, and alcohol or other drug abuse,[5] all of which can be familiar experiences for women who self-injure.

Cutting seems to be the most common method of self-injury, and some researchers find it the method most often associated with prior sexual abuse.[6] A child's age when the abuse first began, the nature of her relationship to her abuser, the type of sexual abuse, the length of time she was abused, and other factors may all influence the frequency and severity of her cutting. If several people were involved who made a ritual of the abuse, or if she was also forced to harm others or had to watch others being harmed, her self-cutting and other signs of emotional distress may be most severe.

Weeks, months, or years of inescapable fear or horror are the background to each act of self-injury. As I talked with women who injure themselves, their childhoods emerged, forming stories that make the need to self-injure understandable. Peggy is one of only two of my informants who does not cut but instead hits and scratches herself. She is the only one whose childhood memories do not include sexual or physical abuse. Peggy grew up having to keep all her feelings to herself. If she expressed even the smallest hint of anger or frustration her mother would walk away, not look at her, and then, while talking with someone else, joke about Peggy's feelings. Because Peggy's father had two jobs and was never at home, Peggy had nowhere to turn with her emotions. She would go to her room, feeling that she had a choice of exploding inside or banging her arm against the bed or her head against the wall. For a while, Peggy's mother also performed a daily ritual of emotional sadism. She would bring her two daughters together and ask Peggy what color lollipop she wanted. Whatever Peggy replied, her sister would say that she wanted one, too. The mother would not look at Peggy but at Peggy's sister and give the lollipop to her, saying louder than words that Peggy's wishes did not matter, that Peggy herself did not matter.

Mary's father repeatedly raped her, and from her fifth year periodically sold her to a friend for use in a lucrative business of child pornography and prostitution. Before a camera, Mary was subjected to unspeakable sexual acts and physical torture. She then had to watch other children be similarly treated. Mary now carries burn scars from childhood torture by a brand, cigarettes, and candle wax as well as later scars from cutting herself. As an adult, Mary once asked her mother if she hadn't thought it strange that Mary would be gone for weeks at a time and all summer long during childhood. Her mother replied, "I figured it was better not to ask."

Erica's mother was a teacher beloved by generations of students. The generosity she showed her students did not carry over to her own children. At home she attempted to own her daughters, leaving Erica feeling powerless and trapped—feelings that now precede Erica's self-cutting. Erica's mother would regularly, but randomly, come up behind Erica and knock the air out of her by hitting her between the shoulder blades and admonishing her to "Stand up straight!" or "Sit up straight!" These surreptitious attacks, which Erica calls her mother's "favorite trick," would occur out of the blue. Erica's mother also frequently gave her enemas. Years later, Erica heard that frequent enemas can be considered a form of rape by proxy, and Erica's self-cutting began to make sense to her.

Barbara's earliest childhood experiences included having her arms and legs tied to the bed while her grandparents and parents inserted objects into her vagina. Sometimes they would drug her and tell her that it was only a dream. Later in life, around age seven or eight, her father showed her "how to make men happy" through fellatio, pretended that she was his girlfriend, and told her that she was "better" than her mother. From her tenth year, the fellatio was replaced by intercourse. When her mother saw what Barbara's father was doing, she, too, sexually abused Barbara. Throughout her childhood, Barbara chronically felt trapped with no way to vent her overwhelming feelings, similar to the way she now often feels before cutting herself. Barbara can never have children because of the internal damage done to her as a child. Nonetheless, she feels lucky. When she sees her family at a wedding or funeral she thinks, How did I ever get out of there alive?

As children, Esther, Karen, and Jane, now mothers themselves, were regularly subjected to family members' sexual assaults. Esther grew up surrounded by violence. As far as she remembers, her father repeatedly raped and physically abused her, including cutting her twice, and a few of her eleven siblings pinched, hit, and whipped her. She also witnessed cutting, pinching, and hitting, some of it evidently in the context of rituals. From Karen's fifth to eighth years, her father stuck his fingers into her vagina and made her suck his penis. He then stopped such abuse but later began subjecting her to obscene provocations by mail and in person, which he was still doing at the time of the interview when Karen was thirty-nine. Like Karen, Jane experienced abuse both as an adult and as a child. Date rape as a young woman reinforced her childhood experiences of being fondled or raped by six boys and men—her stepfather, three brothers, and two neighbors, making both home and neighborhood unsafe yet physically inescapable surroundings for playing, studying, and sleeping.

Escape

. . . .

Barbara: Sometimes if I feel so trapped, like I did as a kid in battering situations, where you feel like you have all these feelings and nowhere to go with them, nowhere to vent them. That's when I resort to cutting in my current life. That is when I think I already got to my max of how much I could tolerate. When I was younger . . . when it got to the point that I couldn't stand to bear the feeling, I would leave my body. And this is just a way of dealing with that overload, I think. I was chronically in a state of stress growing up by all of the abuse I suffered and not being able to tolerate it. Because I think I would have died—I don't know if you can die from feelings, but I would have killed myself probably if I felt it too much.

. . . .

Faced with unbearable events and emotions, a small child rarely kills herself.[7] Instead, she has to find other means of escaping situations in which she is helpless and overwhelmed. Because of her youth and dependency, she cannot flee, and nothing that she can do will alter her circumstances. When there is no other exit, the child's consciousness can protect itself by leaving her body, a process called dissociation.[8] Leaving the body is a psychological statement: "I distance myself from these events." This process is available to us in our earliest years: entering a trance state is one of the few ways an infant can regulate her emotions.[9] It is also the only way a person of any age can numb the effects of abuse while it occurs. Only after the event can a small child scratch at herself or, as she grows older, use razor blades, hammers, food, or alcohol and other drugs to temporarily relieve the lasting effects of abuse by others.

Dissociation is only one of myriad reasons a woman injures herself, reasons discussed more fully in the following chapters. However, some knowledge of dissociation is crucial to understanding certain aspects of self-injury. Because our minds "travel" every day, dissociation is not difficult to comprehend. Daydreaming is a form of dissociation that can routinely take us to a different time and place, with some of us more susceptible to sustained daydreaming than others. The expression "absentminded" reveals how familiar mild forms of dissociation are in our everyday lives. Hypnosis is induced dissociation, often practiced therapeutically for the purpose of temporarily relieving physical pain, just as other types of dissociation provide an escape from physical and emotional pain.

When everyday life involves repeated abuse, dissociation can become appropriately extreme. Instead of being a voluntary play of the mind, extreme dissociation can protect a person's consciousness from actual events taking place and, over time, become involuntary. Long after the actual abuse has ceased, a woman's consciousness may tend to leave her body whenever she experiences stress or anxiety caused by events in her life or by memories, whether conscious or not. This is apparently why physical numbness is often part of the experience of a woman who injures herself.

Mild dissociation can feel strange, but not unbearable. Peggy tells of standing at the copy machine at work, looking around the office and feeling as if she were not there: "I was really in some space ship operating my body by remote control." In a more severe form however, dissociation can be painful: a woman feels physically and emotionally numb, empty, or dead, and describes herself as "unreal" or "gone." She is unable to distinguish herself from other objects, and unaware of the existence of her body. Although the numbness serves to protect her from insufferable emotions, the feelings of separateness and deadness are themselves unbearable, making a woman feel that she is internally disintegrating. Many women who self-injure say that they sometimes do so in order to feel "real" or "alive" again, and to stop the intolerable feelings of dissociation.

Cutting may be the type of self-injury most strongly linked to prior dissociation.[10] Most of the women I spoke with who cut themselves said that the act of cutting never hurt at first, suggesting that they were severely dissociating at the time. When women do feel pain while injuring themselves, they are often relieved, as though the pain were a reassurance that they are "in" their bodies and therefore real and alive.   ›

The Others

People who have experienced rape, physical abuse, combat, torture, or other traumas often speak of dissociation as a sensation of floating above and looking down on their bodies during the traumatic event. Sometimes the floating also occurs in later years during flashbacks of the trauma or just before and during the act of self-injury. Both Edith and Jane described episodes of being up by the ceiling looking down: Jane was looking down on herself in the act of cutting; Edith was in a prolonged flashback, looking down at herself as an infant in mortal terror during one of her mother's physical attacks.

The most thorough way that a child can dissociate from her besieged body is by having her awareness leave the body for stretches at a time, creating a different identity. Some women who self-injure have one or more alter identities who have other names and behave differently. Women who have alter identities sometimes refer to themselves as "multiples," a shortened form of multiple personality disorder, a term once used in diagnosis but now changed to dissociative identity disorder. An alter identity can take over a woman's body from less than an hour to more than a year, and when a woman comes back to herself she often has no memory of that time in her life. Alter identities can embody feelings or protective wishes related to abuse, or embody parts of a woman's identity: a protector from harm, a sexy woman, a terrified infant, a rational adult, an animal, a spirit, and others. One or more of a woman's alter identities may be violent, causing her to be hospitalized because others fear for her safety and for the safety of those around her. At times, the violence is self-injury.

The alter identity can be a child, adolescent, or adult of either sex. The identity's personality and purpose determine what happens when that identity takes over. Some child identities simply want to play, while some want to punish the original person or, perhaps, punish their bodies. Others want to destroy themselves because they were evidently created during abuse and are stuck in childhood, condemned to repeatedly feel as they did while the abuse was occurring. The most severe cutting is sometimes associated with a child identity.[11]

When a woman with multiple identities has periods of amnesia, she knows that an alter identity was in complete charge. Edith, for example, repeatedly cannot remember parts of what happened a few days ago or at her last therapy session. She has completely lost memory of her ninth school year. Esther, however, sometimes cannot control her voice and behavior although she can hear and see what is happening and remembers the situation afterward. She has become an observer of her alter identity's actions, a phenomenon called co-consciousness.

Some adult identities regularly carry out a woman's activities, such as going to work, going to social events, or being interviewed. I was halfway through the interview with Mary when she told me that I was actually speaking with one of her alter identities because Mary no longer talks. An excerpt from this conversation gives a sense of the complexity of multiple identities:

Q: You seem to have been able to separate cutting completely from your working life.
A: Right.
Q: Why do you think you are able to do that?
A: Because somebody else goes to work.
Q: How does that happen?
A: In a way, over the years it's been prearranged. I have an alter that does most of the work activities.
Q: Does she go away when you come home?
A: Not necessarily. She has some other jobs, but for the most part she's the person who goes to work, and she's the person who does more social interaction. In other words, if we're going to a play with some people, she does those types of social interactions. That's what her job is.
Q: So, she takes over when you have to deal with other people?
A: In a lot of circumstances, yes.
Q: Are you aware when this is going on?
A: Yes, I have co-consciousness up to a point, and I'm aware of Cathy.
Q: Her name is Cathy?
A: Yes.
Q: Can you actually feel the change taking place?
A: Yes, if I'm going to work, it's an agreed upon thing, and the shift is made.

Q: Agreed with whom?

A: Agreed inside, between myself and Cathy.

Q: Is Cathy talking to me now?

A: No, I'm Jennifer. I'm the one who is out most of the time in other environments.

Q: I see, but you're a different person than your actual name.

A: Right.

Q: So this is another person?

A: Right. Mary doesn't function at all. Mary is in the system, but Mary stopped functioning a long time ago.

In Mary's case (or the person whom I continue to call "Mary"), her alter identity actually keeps her from cutting herself during working hours. Some adult identities, however, have no agreed-upon function. Instead, they have an unbearable emotion and self-injure as a result. The times when an identity with unbearable emotions has taken over can be alarming for a woman and her caregivers: control over her body is in someone else's hands. A woman can come back to herself and discover new wounds that she does not remember inflicting. As one alter identity said: "I'm cutting Frances's arm. It's my hand though."[12]

Alter identities, therefore, cannot be separated from the experience of self-injury in women who have several identities. Esther, who has numerous alter identities, sometimes hears their voices inside. She knows what they think and what they would do if they could come out, yet she can sometimes keep them inside and maintain control of her actions. Here she gives examples of the ways they both encourage and prevent self-injury:

. . . .

About 10:00 maybe 11:00 A.M., when I have run out of things to keep my mind busy, I start to think about the dreams [I had the night before] and try and figure out what they mean. And sometimes there'll be voices telling me what the different things mean and then I talk back to them — not out loud, they'd lock me up if I did that — I just talk back to them and say, "No that isn't what happened, don't be saying stuff, making up that stuff," and just feeling horrible. Essentially it comes around to feeling horrible that my mind is making up stuff even though I know on one level that I'm not making it up; I know that it's real. Anyhow, they just start going and going and I have this voice of reason in there; her name is Amy and she's a calming influence most of the time. And she will say stuff to me like, "Look at the facts, try not to get so emotional about it, just look at the facts and calm down." And when I do, and I'm listening to all this stuff, I realize that what's going on in the dream and what the voices are saying all makes sense, like a real sick sense, as in vomiting sick. And then I feel a strong urge to cut: one, to silence everyone to make them stop saying those things, and the other, I guess there's also this feeling that I'm bad or even thinking that my grandfather or my uncle could have been involved with people who did bad things to children — and then I get depressed. I guess the depression comes before the cutting. Sometimes if the depression doesn't go away, then there's more cutting. And then I just put band-aids on them if they need band-aids. I don't cut really deep; a few scars, but they're not real deep and they generally go away. Most of the time I don't bleed so much that I need bandages, but after I've cut I seem to get some kind of pleasure from watching little beads of blood connect and look like a little necklace or a chain. I don't know what that's all about. . . .

If I'm driving and I feel an overwhelming urge to do something, that's generally when I feel like driving into a tree, which is more suicidal than self-injury although that is self-injury, too. I dip into my spirituality and I just go, "God, help me. I can't do it alone." That's how I get through driving — and then pull over. "Somebody else drive, *please!*" I first start with just calling out to God and asking for help. And if it still feels awful, then I pull over and I go away. Somebody else gets me home. I don't know how. One of the alters, I think it's probably Amy. She's the oldest.

. . . .

Esther begins her narrative by describing a process that evidently begins during sleep and ends with cutting. Her thoughts or memories of past feelings and events are in the form of alter identities who talk inside her head and interpret her dreams in ways that Esther initially denies, then accepts as the truth. This truth is unbearable, and a downward spiral of feelings begins that must be released through self-cutting.

Esther then describes her temptation to use her car to release her emotions. Overwhelmed by unbearable feelings while behind the wheel, she leaves her body and a lifesaving identity safely drives her home.

Although it may sound as though some identities cause Esther to injure herself while others save her life, Esther disagrees. For her, cutting is a lifesaving act. The harm some identities bring is not self-injury but the memories and feelings they embody from Esther's past abuse at home.

1 *The Last Secret*
Self-Injuring Women Speak

WARNING TO READERS: Some of the personal experiences quoted in this book, especially in chapters one and three, contain graphic descriptions of self-injury that could be upsetting or, perhaps, even trigger self-injury in some self-injuring readers. You may want to pace your reading, skip some passages, and read when you feel protected and can talk about the text with a trusted person.

. . . .

Edith: You know, the feeling is, that if I don't pick at my body and make it bleed, the tension is going to rise, and out of the top of my head is going to pop a volcano. Sometimes as I'm awakening in the morning, I'll find myself scratching at something. But not just scratching the way you'd scratch at an itch, but actually pulling off a scab or scratching at an old wound to make it bleed again. Usually gardening, or at work, some kind of scratch occurs, and then I start at it. I'll pick at the edges to make it bigger, I'll pick at the part that's already there, I'll pull scabs off. Sometimes, I try to stop myself by leaving a band-aid on. So, I'll put on an antibiotic and put a band-aid on it and five hours later I'll take it all off and pick at it again. This is *pervasive.* Even when I get up at night to go to the bathroom, I may scratch at something without thinking, but clearly with the idea of making it bleed. Even as we're talking about it now, the urge is growing inside of me to just pull off this bandage and pick at the scab underneath. Except that I would never do it in front of you. *No one* ever sees me do this.

. . . .

THE SECRECY of Edith's actions is common among women who injure themselves. They divulge self-injury with such caution that family members, friends, and colleagues can live and work with a woman for years without being aware of what she does to her body. Some women are too ashamed even to tell therapists that they repeatedly, secretly injure themselves at home and at work. Self-injury appears to be the most taboo subject to talk about, the last secret a woman is willing to disclose.

In this chapter, the nine women whose childhood abuses were outlined in the preceding pages tell about self-injury, one of the many possible consequences of abuse. They speak the way they do when they are not afraid of speaking. Usually they are afraid. Their secrecy is necessary because these self-injuring women are full participants in society and are constantly among people who would be horrified if they knew. Self-injuring women who disclose can risk being considered incompetent, crazy, sick, evil, perverse, or dangerous, or being involuntarily hospitalized. Therefore, self-injury often becomes a secret as closely guarded in adulthood as their abuse was in childhood. In order to help other women and themselves, they speak here openly about what they do in secret, and tell of the many feelings and thoughts that help explain their actions.

Edith, one of the first women to talk to me about self-injury, pretends to others that nothing is wrong. As a fifty-one-year-old physical therapist with a postgraduate degree, Edith is a respected professional. Edith's work is a part of her life that her friends and colleagues see, yet her secret life has lasted far longer: Edith has been scratching and picking at herself since she was two or three years old. Injuring herself has always seemed so natural that it is hard for her to think or speak of it as something remarkable:

. . . .

As long as I can remember, I have harmed myself. Of course, I never thought of it in those terms, and I never thought of it as being different. But as a kid, my legs would always have an open sore. I remember picking at them—always. I'm not sure that there's ever been a day in my life that I haven't had something open somewhere from picking at it. You can see the scars on my arms from years of picking—and my legs are the same.

. . . .

Many of us remember picking at scabs as children or even as adults, sometimes absentmindedly. Picking is generally only an occasional habit and leaves no scars. However, for Edith and other formerly abused women who pick at their bodies to relieve their emotions, having at least one scratch or open sore to "go after" can feel like a matter of life or death.

. . . .

Edith: I don't want this open sore on my arm, but if I don't have it, I *have* to have one someplace else. There's a scratch on my leg now, but I don't want to go after it either because my legs are so scarred up, and I want to wear shorts in the summer. But I have to have a place somewhere else in order to let the scab on my arm heal. There always has to be something. There's really a feeling that if I didn't have some place to pick that I would die. And I know that's not real, but that's the *intensity*: that I couldn't survive mentally if I didn't have that; that I would go bonkers—lose it all.

. . . .

Edith sometimes picks at scratches and scabs absentmindedly, not realizing what she has done until afterward. She also picks in her sleep and awakens the next morning wondering why she is bleeding. When anxiety or other emotions set off the picking and scratching, the intensity of her self-injury rises. At such times, Edith's picking is purposeful. She can hear herself inside saying, "I don't care what anybody thinks, I'm going to do this; I need to do this; I have to do this." Picking is so automatic that it is hard for Edith to stop and listen to what she feels, but she has discovered that anxiety often builds, an anxiety that seemingly has no object. When I asked her to describe the anxiety, she said:

. . . .

Are you afraid of anything? Snakes, spiders, anything? I mean, just imagine yourself confronted with your worst fear. And that's what it feels like. But it doesn't have a *name*. [I can't say] "I'm anxious about *this*, I'm anxious about *that*." It's just anxiety, unattached to anything specific. It feels like a balloon blowing up inside of me, and it pushes, and pushes, and pushes, and pushes — until it becomes almost intolerable.

. . . .

Picking is a tremendous release for Edith's anxiety, just as it is for other feelings — such as guilt or anger — that she finds intolerable.

Part of the release Edith feels seems to come from the sight or feel of blood, as though the tension were released through bleeding. Edith speaks of blood loss as "taking care" of anxiety, and high anxiety can require more blood than usual. Sometimes, Edith scratches her skin viciously and long, making a wound bleed and letting it bleed. She once gradually lost the equivalent of four units of blood through picking and scratching, alarming doctors who thought she must be bleeding internally. So great is her need for emotional release that Edith sometimes keeps the same wound open for a year or longer and has to use sanitary pads to soak up the blood.

Over the years Edith has become more aware that the actions that seem so natural to her frighten and repulse others; with this awareness has grown her shame and the effort of having to hide self-injury from the world. She feels that she has "this weird secret that I don't want people to know" and says that it is the last confidence she has ever shared with those closest to her. So hidden is her self-injury that for ten years Edith would not discuss it with her therapist. During therapy sessions Edith would mention "picking and scratching" then dismiss them as nothing. This was an easy evasion because Edith's therapist was reluctant to hear about self-scratching and blood. Not until Edith lost large amounts of blood did her therapist realize that "picking and scratching" were major issues.

Clothing usually covers Edith's scars and active wounds, and even when they are visible, most people, she believes, would not guess their cause. If someone asks what happened, Edith, like a battered woman, is prepared: "I cut myself pruning the raspberry bushes" or "I fell and did this." Edith envisions humiliating disgust and rejection if anyone learned the truth: "Oh, how disgusting! How can you do that? Get away from me, I don't want to even see that." Yet, in spite of her shame, Edith sometimes finds herself with scars on her hands. She realizes that she is trying to say something to the world by scarring a visible part of her body: "You see this exterior that looks to you mostly competent and put together, but there's this horrible mess inside. . . ."

Women who injure themselves are sometimes asked, "Doesn't it hurt?" or "How can you hurt yourself like that?" Yet, often a woman feels no pain when injuring herself, suggesting a degree of dissociation from the body. Edith says that there are times when she has tried to pick at something but it has hurt and the pain has stopped her. Yet, when she viciously scratches at herself, it does not hurt. Or, sometimes on one level Edith may be aware of pain, but on another level not at all. Edith thinks that the lack of pain gives her the ability to continue scratching. Most abused women, she believes, have become used to dealing with pain very quickly "by suppressing it and going into [a] trance, or however it is that we've learned to do that."

Edith's picking and scratching are among methods of self-injury almost as diverse as the women who do them, and many women injure themselves in more than one way. Yet, methods of self-injury can serve different purposes for each woman, as well as different purposes at different times for the same woman. Self-hitting is a form of self-injury that can be a barely conscious part of a woman's daily routine. This is true for Erica, a forty-three-year-old editor and writer:

. . . .

Erica: I think there are lots of inconsequential ways that I do things to myself; unconscious ways that I just might think, "Oh! I'm hitting myself again." I often work at home. So I get up in the morning and do the usual kinds of morning things: have breakfast, feed the cat, read the paper, wash the dishes, shower, dress, get to work: turn on the computer, shift gears. I could be talking to somebody on the phone and be sitting at my desk—it seems funny to be describing these things so deliberately when they're so unconscious, you know? I have a metal ruler that I use for my work and I might just sit there and rap it on my arm over and over again with the sharp edge—unconscious little things that I do while I'm talking on the phone. If I play tennis in the afternoon, I have a habit of bashing myself on the knees with my racket, so I have bruises on my knees all the time. That's done specifically when I'm playing poorly. . . . It's not punishment, it's just reminders: "You can do better than this." If I'm in the shower and—you know in the shower you're kind of thinking about things—my thoughts can take a plummet: thinking about something that isn't going well with work or in my personal life. And there's a wooden-handled brush in the shower that, almost without realizing it—probably after the first hit I'm pretty aware of it because it makes quite a sound—but without really thinking about it I'm just hitting. A hundred small things rather than setting out to break my arm.

· · · · · · · · · ·

For twenty-nine years, Erica has been hitting herself as an automatic reaction to the briefest negative emotion such as anger, disgust, or frustration. She says that hitting is a way of "keeping the balance," of staying in touch with herself. It also serves to remind her to do things differently, to change her behavior. When I asked her to give an example of her thoughts while hitting herself, she said, "It sounds ridiculous doesn't it, but you muff a point [at tennis] or something, well? Screwed something up at work?" When I mentioned that it sounded almost like punishment, Erica said, "Yeah, . . . discipline more than punishment." When Erica hits herself, she feels no pain.

Erica remembers that her sophomore year of high school was the first time she realized that someone else might see her bruises. Instinctively, she knew that it was "too dangerous" to let her bruises show. Although she would have welcomed someone asking her how she was hurt, Erica knew that she could not risk an honest reply and that someone else's help could not replace self-hitting.

Erica often gets bruises from playing catcher for a highly-skilled softball team. She puts herself in the path of the ball or of a runner not with a conscious aim of being hurt, but simply because she does not mind being hurt. Her teammates marvel at her "toughness," and she is tough: she does not play with an instinct for physical safety. Erica's willingness to place herself in danger on the softball field resembles other abused women's subtle emotional, physical, or sexual self-injury. Some women neglect their health or basic needs, feeling that they are worthless and not deserving of physical cleanliness, grooming, comfort, or healthful food. For the same reasons, they do not allow themselves to reach goals or to succeed. They may show how much they hate their bodies by ignoring discomfort or pain from overexertion, perhaps leading to serious problems such as nerve damage or a ruptured disk. Erica's playing suggests that her past experiences have encouraged her to see her body as undeserving of protection and as immune to physical pain.

Erica is used to being scrupulously honest. She sets such great store on truth-telling that she once lost a job because of her defense of homosexuality and her revelation of her own lesbianism. For Erica, one of the most distressing aspects of self-injury is that it forces her to lie. Even while taking a strong stand on ethics, Erica has had to break her own moral code by "watching the lie roll off my tongue" about self-injury. Erica was once an active alcoholic, yet even alcoholism was not as important to hide as self-injury. There is no frame of reference for self-injury, she says; she is alone with it. Therefore, Erica maintains what she calls a "little dictionary of lies" even though lying is counter to her values.

While Erica's hitting is a frequent and barely conscious action in response to fleeting thoughts and emotions, another woman can experience self-hitting as seldom and purposeful, at times in response to a powerful need to be punished and make herself suffer. A woman may deliberately beat her body with a hammer or mallet because she is angry with herself and feels that she deserves the pain and the bruises. She may pause because the beating hurts and because part of her does not want to continue. If part of her thinks she deserves more beating, she will pick up the hammer and continue until her need for punishment is appeased. That self-punitive part of her may be a dissociated identity who remembers her own and perhaps other victims' past abuse and now feels responsible and ashamed of both.

When a woman beats her head or arms against the wall, or beats her head with her fists, the hitting may again be deliberate, but the purpose is not necessarily self-punishment. For Peggy, a thirty-four-year-old worker in human services, beating her head releases mounting emotional tension, offering temporary soothing for life's stresses.

Peggy has hit herself since childhood, a time when any expression of her feelings was ignored or ridiculed, making her feel like she would explode inside without some release of her emotions. Nowadays, when she bangs her head, Peggy sometimes feels only self-hatred even though her initial emotion was fury at another person or circumstance. She describes it this way:

. . . .

When everything starts to collide and I feel overwhelmed and I start to hate my house and hate my life and hate my job—something can happen. I [once got] in the car and started the [engine] and got ready to drive away—then I looked at my son and said: "Where's your bag?" He didn't have it [and I went back into the house to get it]. And that was just enough to set me off. I feel it building up and I make faces and I look and feel like I want to *punch* something. But then I feel guilty for being mad. What he did was the trigger, but I realize that what he did in forgetting it was just the last in a long list of things including things that *I* did. And I finally had to release some of it — it's almost like it's a release. So I took the fists of my hands and pounded my head a few times and then looked around and hoped there was nobody there that saw it. Then I [got back into the car and] went off on my road.

· · · · · · · · · ·

Peggy says that sometimes hitting herself is impulsive, but at other times she just thinks about it a lot and tries to stop her thoughts. For Peggy, thinking about it usually does not lead to doing it. Yet, she can be doing chores around the house, not thinking about hitting herself, and something can happen that sets off an overwhelming feeling, sometimes anger. Peggy tries to be prepared for such events because she knows how she reacts to unexpected, strong feelings. She remembers once getting a phone call that now seems unimportant, but at the time "it triggered off a lot of things and I just sort of exploded — the lid blew off" and she hit herself. After such episodes, Peggy feels a bit embarrassed and bad about herself but she also feels less overwhelmed. "It does work, that's the problem with it. If only it didn't work so well."

During periods of her life when she was not hitting herself, Peggy used to deny herself food and call her behavior "dieting." She has never been anorexic, she says, but there have been times when it almost felt good to be hungry. She thinks self-injury is too strong a word for her denial, preferring to call it a way of not being kind to herself. Peggy's method of not being kind may be related to other women's use of food as a form of self-injury: refusing all food as self-punishment, purposely eating to the point of pain, eating or drinking certain foods to cause discomfort, or using laxatives or vomiting after a binge as a way of injuring themselves.[1]

Peggy remarked during our interviews that she has no idea if the things she does to herself are widespread or rare, so secret are they. She thinks that self-injury is at the top of a hierarchy of taboos. Peggy has many friends who have been in therapy, and she feels comfortable talking with them about her depression and medication. But hitting oneself "goes a little bit further" than depression, Peggy finds, so that even among close friends who know of other painful things in her life, very few know about self-injury. "I think that would freak somebody out. Maybe I'm wrong, but I don't tell people." Peggy's therapist once told her that sexual abuse becomes a big secret if the abused person tells no one. Peggy feels that self-injury is like that. "It becomes this barrier, this secret, this thing that I hide." She has other behaviors embarrassing to her, such as twitching in bed or startled jumping, but having someone see her lie in bed twitching would not be as bad as being caught banging her head against the wall: "To me, that's the ultimate of what somebody could see that I would just want to die about."

Once Peggy scratched her arm with her fingernails, leaving three scabs straight in a row that were difficult to explain away. She often thinks about cutting herself but never has, although she has used the tip of a knife to scratch herself, and once scratched "I hate" on her breasts. Peggy's self-hitting leaves no visible traces, and she realizes her good fortune. She speculates that her fear of visible scars helps keep her from scratching herself more often and from cutting herself. Also, as far as Peggy remembers, she was not physically or sexually abused as a child, and her experiences of dissociation are relatively mild—factors that may help protect her from cutting.

Edith and Erica, however, have both cut themselves. To them, cutting feels quite different from picking or hitting. Edith says that self-cutting seems to arise from higher levels of stress and to be more circumscribed than the picking and scratching: she can soon feel "that's enough." Erica says that before she cuts she is incapable of dealing with things and feels that any movement takes great effort, as though she were bound in cotton. Cutting loosens her, makes her able to move again. Erica seems to be describing dissociation, the out-of-body state that often precedes cutting. Such experiences are quite different from the self-hitting that is integrated into Erica's daily life and sometimes seems almost unconscious.

Cutting one's body with a knife or razor can involve a variety of sensations and emotions that sometimes feel stuck in the body, inexpressible except through cutting. The emotions can be so powerful that a woman fears releasing them any other way, or feels that she would kill herself if she could not release them by cutting.

Elizabeth, a twenty-five-year-old typist, tells how feelings related to past abuse by her brother are released in adulthood through self-cutting:

. . . .

Sometimes it will start the night before. Something will happen, maybe a phone call that shouldn't even affect me. Sometimes I need to *find* an excuse to cut because I know it's an addiction, but there always has to be a reason for me to do it. I won't just do it on a great day. So . . . I let the smallest little thing bother me just so that I can say, "I need to cut because *this* happened." I'll wake up the next morning, and I have this nagging feeling that something is wrong. So it's in the very back of my mind: "You're going to cut today." It's like there's somebody in there that tells me I'm going to do it, and I just say:

"Fine." So I'll go through my daily routine. I get up, and real calmly I'll take my shower, I'll eat breakfast — but I'm not really there. It's so weird; I'm just going through the motions, but in the back of my mind I know; I'm almost planning it out: what I'm going to do, when I'm going to do it. And if I have to run errands, I'll run errands.

At a certain time I'll be like, "Alright, now I have to do it, I *have* to go home and do it." . . . I'm so anxious to get home because it's starting to build up and build up, and I know that the time is getting there that I have to do it. I'll drive home and I don't want to talk to anybody. I'll turn my phone off, go right up to my room, lock my door, take out my razor blades and my box of tissues, sit in front of the mirror, take off my sweater (and I just have short sleeves on) — and I look at my reflection for a few minutes. It's almost like I want to do that so that I can know that I have to cut. I look at myself, and at that moment, I hate myself. I'll tell myself, "You're so worthless" because I'm building up to cutting. And then I'll feel it. It's like, "Alright, I'm at the top now, I have to do it *now*." I'll take the razor blade and — I do it really slowly. I'll take it and I'll press it in as deep as I can into the skin, and I'll just go all across my arm. It will start bleeding right away, and I'll just wipe away the blood. Then I'll start again, and this time I'll go deeper. I don't feel pain but I feel — right here in my chest — there's a release. It's like something breaks away; I can almost feel it. I take a deep breath, sit there, and hold my arm up like this and let the blood all come down because I want to see that. It's like I'm bleeding it out of me. But it's still not *enough*. I still need to do it again. So I'll keep going over it and over it and over it until — until I don't feel anything.

And then I'll stop and sit there and admire it. I just sit there and I don't even look at me, I don't look at my face. I just stare at my arm and I look real close at the cut. To somebody else it looks so gross but to me, it looks — good. I sit there and I look at it, and I *like* when it's bleeding. If it stops bleeding too soon, I'll do it again until it bleeds. Because I just have to sit there and watch it bleed. . . . I know this is going to sound crazy but it makes me feel good when I see it, because it makes me feel like, "There it is, this is real, and I'm bleeding it." It also makes me feel like I'm almost acknowledging the pain in the past because sometimes I'll be like, "It wasn't a big deal. I don't know why counselors and people in the hospital are making such a big deal about it. [My brother] came in [to my bedroom], he did what he did. The next day I blocked it." But when I do this, it's almost like, "There we go; there's the physical aspect of it . . . ; I know it's there. I'm not losing my mind. I'm not crazy." . . .

When I'm cutting, I'm always smiling. I feel an inner relief: something is breaking away from my soul; something that I didn't want to be there is being taken out through the cutting. And when I'm done, it's not there anymore. I don't know if I physically smile, but inside I'm smiling. It's so weird because it's like there's somebody else inside of me who initiates the cutting and who enjoys it and likes it. . . .

[When] I watch in the mirror as I do it, I just watch my arm, but I never look at my face. And one night I looked at my face and I almost didn't even recognize it. It was totally — it kind of freaked me *out* — it was totally blank. I was feeling all these things inside, but it was coming out through my arm. But even though I was feeling all these things, when I looked and I saw my face, it was totally blank; it was like I was looking at a stranger. I kind of sat there and studied my face for a few minutes and it was weird because it was like it wasn't *me* I was looking at. . . .

You know, sometimes if I'm trying not to do it but I want to do it, I feel like I'm going to explode inside because I can't deal with the emotions that I'm feeling. I don't know how to deal with my emotions verbally. It's like, "Oh my God! If I don't cut I'm not going to be able to handle it and it's going to get worse and I'll probably kill myself or something." This may be self-destructive, but it's not suicidal and it's not going to kill me. But if I don't deal with these emotions . . . I swear I'll do something drastic. That's how I feel. So I'll cut, and it's gone then. It makes sense to *me*.

And no matter how deep I go, or how large the cut is, it never hurts. I always just feel that something locked inside is coming out through the cutting, and it frees me from it, even though it's only temporary. And right now where I'm at, I would rather keep cutting and getting temporary relief — even though it means that I have to go back and do it a few days afterward — rather than go through all of the pain and feel all of the suffering to get past it.

· · · · · · · · ·

Elizabeth describes an addiction to cutting that has almost taken a life of its own, that requires only an "excuse." In this case, a phone call seems to trigger a response later during sleep, and Elizabeth awakens knowing she is going to cut. Without using the terms "dissociation" or "alter identities," she seems to be describing them when she recounts how she calmly begins the day "not really there" and feeling like she has been taken over: "It's like there's somebody in there that tells me I'm going to do it, and I just say, 'Fine.'" She can hold off until the urge is at its peak, but before she cuts she has to look at her image in the mirror as a reminder of her self-hatred, as though what she is about to do is a punishment for unnamed offenses as well as a release. The moment of release is like surgery: she cuts, blood flows, and something that was "locked inside" breaks away as though it had been cut loose or cut out of her body. The surgery is healing, at least temporarily: "Something that I didn't want to be there is being taken out through the cutting. And when I'm done, it's not there anymore." The cutting is also reminiscent of the longstanding belief that bleeding a sick person releases "bad" blood and heals. Elizabeth seems to literally bleed out her emotions. "I was feeling all these things inside, but it was coming out through my arm." Simultaneously, the act of cutting serves to make her internal pain concrete, believable—something she and others should acknowledge and take seriously. "It makes me feel like, 'There it is, this is real, and I'm bleeding it.'" After the cutting, once again the mysterious "someone" inside Elizabeth makes herself noticed by being pleased and smiling because of the cutting, or by revealing in the mirror an eerie detachment of Elizabeth's face and body from her turbulent consciousness. Elizabeth realizes that she cannot use words to subdue her emotions but that they must be released if she is to remain alive and functional. Cutting is her solution.

Jane, Mary, Karen, and Esther are four mothers in their thirties and forties who also work outside the home. Secretly, they cut themselves. Although self-cutting is a commonality among these four, each woman's experiences with it differs. Jane, a treasurer and married mother of three, finds that the need to cut sometimes simply seems to be there, as though planted in her mind during sleep.

. . . .

My two oldest sons leave between 6:30 and 7:00 A.M., and I get my youngest one up, and he leaves a little before 8:00. And during that whole time period, I would have in the back of my mind that . . . I was planning on cutting myself. Usually for some reason I get in my head that I need to be punished, or sometimes I feel like I've got poison running through my body and by cutting I'll release the poison. And logically I know that's not true, but it gets into some part of my brain, and I can't let go of it. I have the really strong feeling that if I cut I'll feel better, and sometimes it actually does feel better for a while.

I get into the tub and usually I cut my arm inside the elbow. The last time I cut there, I was disappointed because I wasn't able to get as deep as I wanted to. I couldn't seem to get the amount of blood. I was struggling to get deeper—I don't make long cuts, I make small, but deep, cuts. I don't know how long I was there, but the whole time I was doing it, I had this argument going back and forth in my head: part of me encouraging myself to go ahead and do it and to go deeper, and part of me saying how stupid it is. Sometimes what I'm thinking is, "I can't believe I did it again. It's so stupid. When's it going to stop?" Other times, what's in the forefront of my mind is whether or not I got a good bleed; how soon I can do it again.

. . . .

It is strange, Jane says, how much pleasure she gets from watching herself bleed. The longer she goes without cutting herself, the more blood must flow to release her feelings. Afterward, Jane sometimes feels guilty and upset for having cut herself, and her resulting embarrassment and humiliation are hard for her to bear. This is often the case among women like Jane who discuss self-injury with their therapists and are trying to stop. Jane tends to repeatedly cut over a previous scar so that she does not have many scars on her body. When she goes out, she can easily excuse her long sleeves because of fibromyalgia, a socially acceptable condition requiring warmth to prevent joint achiness. The most difficult task is hiding a new cut from her husband who knows about and tries to discourage Jane's self-injury. This conjugal secrecy is so important to Jane that dread of his discovery increases her control over cutting during the summer months when long sleeves are uncomfortable and more difficult to excuse.

During periods of cutting it feels unsafe to Jane to let her feelings out, as though they were uncontrollable animals too dangerous to release. Her emotions then bury themselves and Jane feels nothing, not even the seemingly harmless pleasure or discontent that are usually part of everyday life. Jane seems to be describing the emotional numbness often found among those who have experienced past trauma. In order to appear "normal," Jane used to act the emotions she thought the most appropriate. Other abused women sometimes also simulate gaiety or tearfulness when they feel only empty and dead. Ironically, acted emotions may look quite exaggerated, leading a woman's companions or therapists to suspect her of "putting on an act," which indeed she is.

Like most women with whom I spoke, Jane at first feels no pain when cutting, although pain may come after cutting awhile and be a signal to stop. Self-cutting is often painless because physical numbness is part of the state of dissociation that can precede cutting. Yet, for some women, self-cutting is sometimes or always immediately painful, and the pain is an important component: it feels gratifying, like a release or punishment. Even when cutting is painless, a woman can feel pain immediately when hitting or burning herself, and the pain itself relieves her emotions. Constant pain may help her get through each day: cutting the soles of one's feet causes pain with every step; inserting a safety pin into the arm hurts with every arm movement. Pain can be one of the objectives of self-injury, perhaps release or distract from emotional pain, perhaps to keep a woman "in her body," perhaps for self-punishment.[2]

. . . .

Jane: There have been times when, instead of cutting my arm, or my ankle, when I've cut inside my vagina, or done other things to cause pain: inserting a stiff brush into my vagina. For a while I was using a bottle brush that was fairly stiff — and sometimes leaving it in there so that I felt pain through most of the day. . . . I've wrapped elastics around my nipples, and I would place thumbtacks so that the points were going into my nipples and I would either use tape to hold them in place or wear a tight bra and leave them like that for a few hours, intentionally rubbing them at times to increase the pain.

. . . .

Jane offered no explanation for her occasional need for pain, and the topic was so upsetting to her that we had to quickly change the subject. Other women, however, say that when pain is used for self-punishment and in-volves hurting the nipples or vagina, they are sometimes responding to sexual thoughts or to feeling sexually attracted to someone. They may be simultane-ously responding to memories of rape or other sexual abuse and to any sex-ual arousal they may have felt during the abuse. Their past experiences have taught them that sexual arousal is bad and that the body must be punished for it, especially those parts of the body that "caused" anguish and shame during childhood. Painfully twisting and pinching nipples and thinking self-punitive obscenities like "Who do you think you are, you blank, blank, blank?" are their penance.

For other women who, like Jane, were sexually abused as children, sex itself can offer ways of being injured and self-injury can bring sexual pleasure. Be-cause sexual abuse can arouse a child even while causing pain, sexual arousal and pain can become intertwined and remain so in adulthood. A woman may find that she gets sexual pleasure from being cut by someone else and perhaps perform sadomasochistic sex scenes in order to have opportunities for this type of arousal. At times, sadomasochism may be like a repetition of childhood abuse with the important difference that a woman now feels in control. Other ways of experiencing similar sensations are to invite or submit to bondage or to participate in pornographic films, an industry that repeats, for large profits, many self-injuring women's childhood experiences at home.

As a child, Mary was periodically sold for use in such films. Now, she is a technology manager for a major communications company and divorced mother of two. She also cuts her arms, breasts, stomach, and thighs. Sometimes she does not even realize she is cutting until after the fact; at other times she is under great stress or feels "so much emotion" — or emotional pain — that she has an uncontrollable urge to cut herself. The need for relief and to see blood is so strong that Mary will struggle intensely with the urge to cut herself but not be able to find another way of coping. Mary calls cutting a "safety valve" to release her emotions, just as picking is for Edith and hitting is for Peggy. Here Mary describes a typical working day:

. . . .

The alarm goes off and I get up. I shower, brush my teeth, take my medication, get dressed. I don't usually eat breakfast at home so I go out and get in the car. I usually pick up coffee at a Seven-Eleven and take it into work with me. I go into work and I'm either preparing for a meeting or preparing documentation or running a meeting. I go through the workday and . . . I pretty well block everything else out. I stay very focused at work. When the workday ends I come home and have some dinner. I read quite a bit, so I'll do some reading.

The nighttime is when agitation really starts. If I am having a bad day, I go to bed around 11:00 P.M., and I can go to sleep right away, but I usually wake up in a couple of hours and I have a lot of nightmares. Sometimes I wake up and I can come out of the nightmares and sometimes I don't come out of them; I'm still half in and half out. I can have panic attacks, and on a really bad night, the panic attacks won't go away. I try to be very contained and curl up and be very quiet and still [to] make the panicky, agitated feelings go away. But sometimes it goes on and on and on. These are the danger times, when cutting becomes very hard not to do, and that is the time when cutting is a way to release some of the anxiety and some of the pain. I will reach such a point of agitation that I will either have something in the house, or I have gotten up in the middle of the night and found someplace that was open and bought razor blades and come home and cut. That helps relieve a lot of that anxiety. There are other times. If I'm going through a bad spell, I can be triggered very easily into bad memories. I get real vivid memories that will become a focus and I can't seem to get away from them. . . . That's kind of bad too and can result in cutting.

[Afterward], I usually want to go to sleep. Even if it is the daytime or whatever, I feel so relieved and so relaxed that I just patch up whatever needs to be patched up depending on how extreme it is, and go lie down. It really feels good; there is almost a pleasure in it. It's almost like a relaxation that comes — that kind of pleasure, like if you were very tense and all of a sudden your body relaxed and it kind of exhales. It is that kind of feeling.

          . . . .

For Mary's states of acute anxiety, cutting is her main resource. Nighttime, in bed, is often the most difficult time for Mary whose self-injury, like Jane's and Elizabeth's, seems sometimes triggered by a process that occurs during sleep. Mary, who has several efficient alter identities to help her through the day, cannot escape her feelings and memories at night.

Self-cutting makes Mary feel that she has no control. Every time she has a fresh wound to hide, she feels like a failure. Usually, she covers the many scars on her arms with long sleeves because of the embarrassment she would feel if anyone saw them. Some of Mary's scars are simply faint white lines on her skin, which she sometimes does not mind revealing. Most people say nothing, Mary finds, and if a question is asked, she keeps talking about something else as though she had not heard. She believes that most people do not really want to know what lies behind scars and that politeness also prevents adults from commenting. Like many scarred women, Mary does not mind if scars show as long as no one comments or stares. Nonetheless, Mary is careful to keep large scars covered. If all of Mary's scars could speak, listeners might close their ears in double horror: while some of Mary's scars are self-inflicted, others were inflicted by adults during scenes of childhood torture.

Mary also has a deeper sense of secrecy related to her scars: She is ashamed of what happened to her as a child, and because of this shame she cannot look at her psychiatrist and talk about the childhood abuse she suffered. Instead, she writes the unspeakable acts in her journal for him to read. Mary thinks that because she cannot speak of the past, pressure builds that must be released by cutting.

Mary does let others injure her in a way perhaps similar to sadomasochistic sex. She realized this when she had herself tattooed:

. . . .

The first tattoo I ever got in my life was six months ago and I now have four of them. What I have discovered is, I was using that as a way to do cutting in an acceptable fashion. And I have since found out that it can be a common practice. It feels really good. I have a tattoo on each one of my breasts, on the higher portion of it, and I use them to cover up some old scars, not from me but from stuff that was done to me. You feel the same sense of the blood and the cutting when you have the tattoo done.

          . . . .

For Mary, the prick of the tattoo needle provides release and sometimes sexual arousal. As Mary notes, it has the additional advantages of being socially acceptable and of covering scars from her past abuse.

Karen is a human services manager and married mother of two. Since high school, she has been secretly cutting herself with razor blades: "I just felt a need to feel this release. I've done it ever since whenever I felt really stressed out." It started as a fascination with the blood, and with seeing how she would feel and if it would hurt. Later on, it became irresistible and she had to keep doing it.

Like Mary, Karen finds that one of the most distressing things about self-injury is the feeling that it is inevitable. She is never sure when she is going to give in to an urge and always has to be on guard, never completely trusting herself. Sometimes her psychiatrist will suggest a new medication, giving Karen hope. When she nonetheless resorts to cutting again, the disappointment is humiliating: "Oh, God! I've done it again; I just can't believe that I've done it again."

Karen feels ashamed when she looks at her body. She has considered having cosmetic surgery to erase scars she finds ugly, upsetting, and a constant reminder. But then, something about her scars makes Karen feel secure, as though scars were a proof of pain without having to speak about it; a guarantee of help without having to ask for it. Yet, Karen does not want to show her scars because of the shame attached, so the scars that reveal her past must themselves be hidden. They are a proof of her pain even when no one else can see them.

When her father does something obscene and provocative, Karen cuts her vagina. Her father, who stuck his fingers into her vagina and made her suck his penis when Karen was five to eight years old, now sends Karen photographs of his penis. Karen thinks that she cuts her vagina at such times because her father has destroyed part of her sexuality: "I don't like that part. I want to hurt it."

Cutting is the only way Karen injures herself, and she resorts to it every few months. Sometimes, though, she is able to stop herself, especially if there are no sharp objects around. At other times she cuts from an overwhelming urge because she does not know what else to do with the tension inside. When she is alone, her thoughts can take over and she will think of killing herself, family members, or her therapist to "get back" at people who have hurt her. She releases these aggressions by injuring herself. Cutting immediately relieves the initial tension but also triggers additional negative feelings because Karen knows that there will be "repercussions" if she tells her therapist, who will ask if she has injured herself, or if her husband notices the fresh wound. Karen then feels guilty, ashamed, and disappointed that she was not able to stop herself. When Karen cuts, she continues until she begins to feel pain.

. . . .

Karen: The last time I cut myself really badly, I felt that people weren't hearing me. And I felt very anxious about my situation and that people didn't realize how bad it was for me. So, I cut my arm with a razor blade and then my first response was that I was scared. But as time went on I felt sort of a sense of relief that I'd done it and that people would notice.

In order to do it, I have to project this hate thing on myself. I tell myself, "You're horrible, you deserve. . . ." Or sometimes if I'm angry at someone, if I'm angry at my husband I'll say things to myself like, "All right, I'm going to show you; I'm going to pay you back," and then I'll cut *myself.* It's anger misdirected, a lot of depression . . . and a feeling of helplessness about something; or oftentimes a feeling of gigantic loss. Somehow I have to punish myself for that. I don't understand why, but that's the way it comes out.

What happens the most is, I sense that I'm going to lose something, whether it's a relationship or it's just something that I need. I sense that I'm going to be abandoned, and I can't bear the pain. So I do this. . . . I could be talking to my therapist and feel that she's decided that she's not going to be seeing me anymore. I realize that I get paranoid about that but I haven't really dealt with it. I'm always going back and forth with "I don't need this person; I'm going to end it," and then feeling "Oh, my God, I can't live without this; I'm going to lose it," and then wanting to hurt myself, and being confused about what's real and what isn't.

I also get [to] feeling bad just simply by listening to music that reminds me of a certain time in my life. I can start to feel depressed about it to the point where I'm in a downward spiral. It can happen fairly fast if I'm alone with nothing to distract me.

Sometimes the cutting is erotic; it evokes erotic feelings. That's odd, but that's the way it is. When I'm cutting or just before I cut, I sometimes think erotic thoughts. It's not really like arousal but it's similar to it. The cutting is like a release. And it's not every time it happens like that, but sometimes.

. . . .

Karen's words reveal the variety of thoughts and emotions in one woman that can precede cutting: frustration, anger, depression, helplessness, self-hatred, erotic feelings, a fear of impending loss, and a need to ask for help. Karen's thoughts and emotions may appear to be as inexplicable as Mary's panic, or Jane's "poisoned" blood and need for punishment, but only because their roots probably lie in the past and are not consciously attached to the childhood events that would help explain them.

Just as Karen's emotions vary, so do all three women's descriptions of cutting because each woman's reasons for cutting are shaped by her past and present experiences and emotional makeup. Experiences with cutting can differ from day to day and over the years. A single cutting episode can last half a minute or take half a day of intermittent cutting behind closed doors. A woman can cut to return to her body and to leave her body; she can cut when she is angry and when she feels nothing; she can cut to punish herself and to avoid suicide; she can begin cutting herself around puberty, stop at eighteen, and start again at forty-five; she can cut for thirty years, then stop in her forties or fifties.

In spite of such variations, most cutting—and perhaps picking—seems to have at least one commonality: blood.[3] The sight of blood gives release, no matter what the initial emotions. At times, the greater the emotional turmoil, the more blood must flow to appease it. The sensation of warm blood flowing can be as important as the sight of it. Blood's meanings are still something of a mystery. Perhaps the act of bleeding proves to women who are dissociating that they have bodies and are alive. Some women refer explicitly to the life-giving effect of cutting and seeing blood as a release from dissociation: "I feel my life come back into me"; "I make myself feel something"; "I could see that I was real." The amount of blood may sometimes signify that a cut was severe enough to bring relief. Some women also need to do something with their blood, such as taste or suck it, preserve it in bottles, or let it "speak" by writing or painting with it. One woman I talked with provided an explanation for her own experiences with blood: she sometimes tastes her blood to make sure that it is truly blood, proving that it was her living body she had just cut. Perhaps blood saved in bottles serves as proof of life for some self-injuring women, analogous to the life-giving connotation of bottled blood for transfusions. Bottling blood could also be a reenactment of rituals experienced during childhood.

Blood is not the only important component of self-cutting, however; some women find it equally important to see the flesh of a deep cut open the second before blood appears: that sight is part of the release. Even the ritual of cutting—taking out the knife or razor blades, disinfecting the skin with alcohol before cutting, and cleaning the blood away afterward—can provide some satisfaction.

In contrast to other forms of self-injury, cutting oneself may be confined to the menstrual years in many women, beginning around menarche and subsiding during the premenopausal or menopausal years,[4] if it has not been overcome sooner. This rhythm may be related to the cycles of estrogen and progesterone that can increase a woman's sensitivity to stress and her susceptibility to depression and anxiety.[5] The same holds true for the monthly patterns of self-injury that some women detect.

Esther, a married mother of two, is a security station operator during the day and a sales associate in the evenings. She has been cutting herself for thirty years. From time to time, she pinches her nipples and, when she has promised her therapist not to cut, hits herself. Like Jane, Mary, and Karen, Esther usually cuts herself in response to unbearable sensations or emotions. Yet, while preparing a meal, cutting open a fish or other food can trigger an urge to cut into her own flesh and do it more deeply than usual. This is similar to some women's experiences that any accidental injury to the body feels like an invitation to make the bruise bigger or the cut bloodier.

When she was five, Esther's father once cut her around her ankle with a jackknife in what Esther thinks may have been part of a ritual. As an adult Esther once cut herself with a jackknife on the same place, in what seems to her a reenactment of her father's abuse: "It was like a symbolic thing. . . . What was going through my mind was anger, and there were these words: 'Never going to run away from me again, are ya.' It was almost like it was the exact same thing." Such reenactments are a part of many self-injuring women's experiences, perhaps especially among those whose abuse occurred in a ritual context.[6] At times, a reenactment can be an unconscious way of retrieving the memory of past trauma and a nonverbal way of telling about it. Another type of reenactment occurs when a woman does not repeat the same abuse but feels that because her body was once abused, it should continue to be injured in some way: "If nobody else is going to do it, now I have to" can be one among many simultaneous reasons for self injury.

Esther also leaves knives or fishing hooks lying in a boat and steps on them; "tests" with her arm to see how hot a bonfire is; and uses kitchen knives carelessly. She has learned that being accident-prone can itself be a form of self-injury. Other women who are aware of their accident-proneness speak of trying to catch a falling hot iron, dropping heavy objects on their feet, and falling down. Even some industrial and traffic accidents may be forms of severe self-injury.[7] These events are not consciously planned or carried out with the goal of self-injury and can, therefore, be a secret even to the woman herself. Esther has had such "accidents" but realizes that her resulting injuries are not truly accidental.

. . . .

You know, it's funny how quickly you can tell yourself that it's an accident but in the back of your mind you're saying, "I don't know if it really was an accident or not." You can just tell yourself so quickly, "Oh, it was an accident, it was an accident," and you believe it of yourself right away! So, it's hard to tell sometimes if it really was an accident or not. I mean, just like [with] a child who has a lot of accidents, you'd be suspicious that the parents were abusing her. It's like saying, "Too many accidents for this to be accidental."

. . . .

Esther considers herself fortunate because her husband is not abusive. Childhood sexual, physical, or emotional abuse or neglect can make a woman feel worthless, ugly, powerless, and incompetent[8] — feelings that make her a target for abuse in adulthood and that discourage any thoughts she may have of escape. Esther realizes that having an abusive partner can be a method of self-injury — of continuing to be a victim of the violence a woman grew up with, the only kind of "love" her body knows.[9]

Esther also eats to soothe herself, a behavior she shares with the majority of women with whom I spoke. Like self-injury, food can temporarily numb women's emotional pain, a fact confirmed by countless women who use food as a tranquilizer or anesthetic. Food soothes in many ways. For one woman, having food in her mouth keeps away bad thoughts or feelings that return immediately when she stops eating. For another, constantly nibbling comes from a craving forever unsatisfied. But the taste of food also feels good; eating keeps her hands busy so that she does not pick at herself; and being "about a hundred pounds overweight" protects her from men and, perhaps, from her own sensations and emotions.[10] A third woman may binge-eat and take laxatives to keep her weight down, swinging back and forth between periods of cutting herself and periods of binging and purging, as though one were a substitute anesthetic for the other. Esther's eating seems to come from the need for a milder and more fleeting anesthetic than the alcohol and other drugs she used to take.

One of Esther's greatest fears is being surprised by a question about scars without being able to think of a quick, smooth, believable response. She never wears dresses or skirts because her legs are scarred, including a bad scar from the childhood injury her father inflicted. Yet, Esther's secrecy is partial and reluctant. On hot days, she sometimes wears shorter sleeves to work. Esther considers this a big step forward: "I could cover them, but they'd still be there. The problem that's causing them is still there, so why should I cover it up — to make other people more comfortable?" When a patron at Esther's evening job once asked about the scars and provided an alibi — "Do you work with animals?" — Esther simply said, "No, it's not from working with animals," and went on to tell about her day job as a security station operator. "You can guess car accident or anything else you want; I might have been doing rose bushes or something. . . . But I didn't feel like I owed her an explanation and I'm hoping that I can keep that sense of privacy for myself—they don't need to know." Esther has found a mixture of disclosure by revealing some of her scars, and of secrecy by not feeling obliged to explain them. She thinks that truthfulness could encourage her recovery. Esther wants to sometimes be able to say, "This isn't from my cat or my dog, this is from my knife," and be understood when she explains that shame or anger caused the cuts.

Barbara has gone even further than Esther in truth-telling. She is determined to help shake self-injury's hold on her by speaking more openly about it. Yet, Barbara has more to hide than many self-injuring women because of the variety of ways she self-injures, lets herself be injured, or intentionally risks injury.

Barbara, a thirty-eight-year-old social worker, has been injuring herself for seventeen years. Cutting is her main method, but she uses different ways of cutting depending on her emotional state. Sometimes she simply needs to see blood and a scratch will suffice. At other times, she wants to mutilate or even eviscerate herself. This frightening need results in deep cuts, injuring tendons and muscles, and requiring stitches and other care. During such acute emotional states, she sometimes burns herself—pressing a hot iron or other heated metal object against her skin—instead of cutting, fearing for her life if she allows herself to use a knife or razor. Burning is currently not a frequent form of self-injury for Barbara, a statement true of all the women I interviewed, although self-burning may be prominent in some women. Instead, self-burning is an occasional thing for Barbara, but was done more often in the past. She once switched entirely to burning for a while after she miscalculated the severity of one cut and her therapist taught her to be wary of inadvertent suicide.

Barbara sometimes cuts herself because she feels that she is floating in space and needs to anchor herself. At other times, she cuts because she wants to escape her feelings or because she simply wants to see blood. During her everyday routine, Barbara may soothe herself by superficially scratching with any pointed object at hand; by letting herself be scratched by her playful cat; by eating; or by pulling at her hair, sometimes unintentionally pulling some out.

Barbara gets a feeling of satisfaction by having things sticking into her and seeing them coming out of her body. For a while she regularly sold her blood to a blood bank, liking this way of having needles stuck into her in a socially acceptable fashion. Like many women who injure themselves, Barbara once bore her otherwise unbearable emotions with the help of alcohol, heroin, and cocaine. Having needles in her arm was part of her addiction to the intravenous drugs.[11] The ritual of preparing the injection and cleaning the needles afterward were also part of her addiction.

When Barbara overcame her drug addictions, she found herself doing other things to appease her emotions. Besides increasing her cutting, she began compulsively shopping. Sometimes she would also compulsively shoplift or drive recklessly, feeling that taking risks would get her adrenaline flowing so that she could feel alive and in the present rather than physically and emotionally numb and absent from her body. Even in less acute emotional states, Barbara sometimes incorporates risks into her life by standing at the edge of a cliff to look at a view, or by jumping from a high place into an unfamiliar lake before swimming.

In spite of these signs that Barbara has little instinct to preserve her body from harm and extinction, she considers that she actually has a strong will to live — otherwise, she would not still be alive. She thinks that all of her actions, including self-injury, are forms of self-medication to temporarily appease her emotions. She is fighting hard to free herself from all self-harmful addictions.

Barbara thinks that self-injury is the most socially ostracized relief from mental distress, far more unacceptable than using alcohol or food. Women who injure themselves, she says, are seen as the "lowest of the totem pole." Consequently, like almost every woman with whom I spoke, Barbara has her own repertoire of lies, some of them quite elaborate: "I was weatherizing my windows for the winter and fell through the window," a lie that accounts for many scars at once, or "I was cutting linoleum for the kitchen counter and the blade slipped," to explain a recent gash.

In the past, Barbara went to great pains to hide her scars by trying to be careful where she cut, by clothing, and by counting the days it would take a cut to heal before a doctor's appointment. She has also worn an elastic bandage and pretended to have a sprained arm. Even now, Barbara usually wears long sleeves and long pants to hide her scars, partly because she works in the mental health field and wants to be viewed as a supervisor or fellow staffperson, not as a client. Yet, Barbara now sometimes lets old scars show and recently has begun giving flippant answers to questions — "I had a run-in with a straight-edged razor blade" — and has also occasionally given truthful responses. New scars, however, are hidden because they are "slips" and feel shameful. It is important to her that revealed scars be old ones, part of the past.

Gradually revealing self-injury is frightening for Barbara because it was always such a secret thing. She is coming out about it as part of an attempt at truthfulness about her life, including incest, alcohol and other drug addictions, and her own sexual preference of lesbianism: "I just don't want to live in a closet of any sort." Barbara thinks that keeping secrets is unhealthy, and she associates secrets with her parents and other family members. She is recovering from self-injury and can reveal it more easily because it usually feels like part of the past. As part of her recovery process, Barbara purposely tells the truth about cutting even when a questioner offers her an opportunity to lie: "Did you fall through a window or something?" "No, I cut myself with a razor blade." "Do you shave your arms?" "No, I intentionally did it."

Barbara's new openness is a part of her therapy. and a result of it. For the first seven years of therapy, she was too ashamed even to tell her therapist about her past abuse. She felt like she was "dirty" and should be killed because of her incestuous experiences as a child. She has learned to talk about incest with her therapist and thinks that therapy has helped her see incest as something that happened to her, not something that was her fault; therefore, she need feel no shame about it. Similarly, she now knows that she is not a "bad person" because she cuts: "It's just a syndrome that I fell into."

Barbara does still wish that she had no scars, that they would all fade away, or that she could afford to obliterate them with cosmetic surgery. Yet, at times, they comfort her. She looks at them and charts her progress: "Look at all you have been through, and look where you are now." Barbara compares her changing attitude to someone who first rejects and dyes her gray hairs, then proudly reveals them as landmarks of a long life, experience, and wisdom. Because revealing scars selectively is part of Barbara's overall "coming out," she does not want to have to hide them or hide anything else, but will do so out of practicality—to get a job, for instance—not out of shame. They are a part of who she is, a road map of where she has been, her battle scars.

As these nine women show, self-injury is a highly versatile, secret reaction to diverse states of mind that can often be traced back to childhood abuse. No list of self-injury's functions can be considered complete, but the following summary of the functions mentioned on the preceding pages, as well as other functions,[12] may help reveal self-injury's complexity:

1. to release emotions, whether absentmindedly, as sometimes in daily skin-picking or -hitting; explosively, as in sudden, rageful self-hitting or -cutting; or purposefully, after anticipation and planning
2. to calm turbulent, racing thoughts
3. to discipline, punish, or show hatred and disdain for oneself, one's body, or a specific body part
4. to return to the body after feeling distant from it or unreal
5. to feel distant from the body's thoughts, feelings, and memories
6. to see blood

7. to release poison perceived as running through the body like blood
8. to feel pain
9. to avoid suicide
10. to avoid frightening feelings
11. to stop flashbacks or intrusive, vivid memories
12. to stop the internal voices of alter identities
13. to make internal pain concrete and visible to oneself
14. to reveal internal pain to others without using words
15. to ask for help without using words
16. to tell about past abuse without using words
17. to keep oneself from using words to tell about past abuse
18. to prove to oneself that past experiences were true and abusive
19. to satisfy the feeling that it is "right" to abuse one's own body because it always has been abused
20. to reenact scenes of past abuse
21. to make the outside look the way the inside feels
22. to prevent being hurt by someone else
23. to obey intrusive memories or flashbacks of commands to self-injure given during childhood ritual abuse
24. to communicate a warning from one identity to another in women with multiple identities
25. to recreate the confusion of feelings learned in childhood that:

    closeness and pain are inseparable
    trust and punishment are inseparable
    sexual arousal and being "bad" are inseparable
    sexual arousal and pain are inseparable

The following chapter discusses the pathways linking these functions to past abuse.

2 From Childhood Abuse to Adult Behavior

LINKS BETWEEN childhood experiences and adult behavior are subjects of research that may help explain the internal logic of self-injury. Studying a child's experiences includes assessing how adult caregivers speak to, behave toward, and care for a child, as well as the opportunities a child has to safely explore her or his surroundings. A child's brain develops through the activities of nerve cells called neurons, activities partly determined by genetic codes inherited from parents. Yet, a child's experiences—including abuse—also affect brain development.

Debates continue about the role of genetic inheritance (nature) versus the role of experience (nurture) on brain development and, subsequently, on our feelings and behaviors. Research shows that nature and nurture interact: we genetically inherit our brain's basic structures, but both genetics and our experiences determine the patterns in which neurons connect to one another.[1] It may be possible, some researchers assert, to construct *brain-maps*: configurations of neurons that correspond to patterns of experience.[2] The maps are not static but change continuously as a result of new experiences. In this way, what once was learned from negative experiences can remain throughout life to affect our thoughts and behavior, but can also often be unlearned through new insights and experiences, such as the experience of establishing positive relationships with others, including therapists.

Overwhelming, inescapable experiences, called *trauma*, may alter the brain's development in ways that can be detected by brain imaging techniques. Some research suggests that childhood sexual abuse is associated with changes in brain volume.[3] This alteration in size may be the result of the effects of abuse on hormones such as cortisol, catecholamines, opioids, and serotonin that are secreted during stress and affect brain development.[4] These hormones—known as *stress hormones*—are also implicated in changes in the functioning of certain areas of the brain.[5]

Animal studies suggest that early, severe disruptions in a child's ability to attach to a loving, protective person also cause lasting changes to the brain.[6] Such emotional trauma can be inadvertently caused by shuttling parentless newborns from one institution or foster home to another so that they are not adopted until after six months of age. Later, their many problems often include repeated self-injury and the inclination to put themselves in physical danger. Being touched and cuddled as an infant and having consistent adult support in our early years seem crucial in helping us regulate emotions and responses to stress.[7]

Repeated abuse during childhood may leave the limbic system of the brain, an area involved in anger and other intense emotions, with highly excitable nerve cells — a process called *kindling.*[8] In addition, the sympathetic nervous system and brain cells in the locus ceruleus — the brain's "alarm center" — react to uncontrollable stress in ways that appear to be similar whether the stress was combat on a battlefield or abuse at home.[9] Researchers are currently studying various types of chemical imbalances induced by repeated trauma. Such imbalances keep the body's stress hormones at continuously high levels[10] and may later be reactivated by the normal stresses of life, causing a woman to respond volatilely to everyday events. A woman can experience this excitability as chronic anxiety; negative thoughts; or as intermittent, explosive emotion. Some women injure themselves repeatedly in response to seemingly minor stresses, such as a disappointment or quarrel. A woman who self-injures seems to react to many stresses as though she were reliving the original trauma.[11] Therefore, no stress is minor for her, and her life is full of what she perceives as traumatic situations.

During traumatic abuse, the body may secrete soothing chemicals, called endorphins, that numb physical pain and reduce panic,[12] temporarily ending the child's physical and emotional distress. These painkillers also play a role in keeping the person from storing her experience in verbal memory,[13] although she may store it as images, sensations, or feelings. Thus, after the trauma, especially if abuse is repeated over time, a child will not be able to say, "Yesterday, my father tied me to a bed and raped me." Instead, years later, she may repeatedly feel that she cannot move properly, as though her arms and legs were tied, and not understand why she feels this way.[14] She may suddenly feel that past abuse is happening now, yet not know why such flashbacks occur. She can have attacks of panic, multiple fears, and periods of unexplainable anxiety. Actually, she is remembering past abuse in every way except words, but she cannot place these memories in their context. Traumatic abuse has locked her memories into her body, where they can create overwhelming pressure and make her unable to integrate thoughts, feelings, and memories into coherent consciousness. These mute memories can, years later, become insistent and temporarily break down her ability to function normally.

Eventually, dissociated memories may enter verbal consciousness yet continue to cause psychological distress and be extremely painful to recall, painful to the point of suicide:

. . . .

Edith: I did not remember [the trauma]. I'm forty-nine, and I started to get memories back when I was forty-two or forty-three. . . . All I knew when I first went into therapy is: "My life is not good; every year I have these terrible depressions in the fall. I've been doing band-aid therapy, feeling a little bit better, but I don't want to do that anymore. I want to find out." Well, it took me eight years before the memories even started to come back. And that was before the term "survivor" was even out there, when posttraumatic stress disorder belonged only to Vietnam vets. So, I started to have memories. It's taken me a long time, and I'm still uncovering memories. They only come when I'm ready to deal with them . . . and sometimes, that means barely deal with them. . . .

My mother died five and a half years ago, and the fall after my mother died is when I started having whole memories. Up to that point I'd had memory fragments and I knew enough from having them for several years that there had to be some truth to them about my father. But when my mother died, all of a sudden I got *inundated* with memories. I had to take time off from work—I was throwing up memories.

. . . .

The act of self-injury may reactivate endorphins.[15] The body produces endorphins in response to many different stressors, such as the physical stress of running, extreme emotional stress, or the stress of injury such as surgery or an accident. Such internal chemicals can reduce anxiety, rage, aggression, and depression.[16] Animal studies suggest that the prolonged stress of childhood abuse causes the body to respond to subsequent stresses with an increase in soothing chemicals that can produce dependence and withdrawal symptoms.[17] This might help explain why some women say that self-injury has become an addiction. As Edith says:

. . . .

Picking is like doing an endorphin kick: bang! And eating isn't. The eating only works as long as I'm doing it; it's not that it has a lasting effect. Picking at something really is a lasting drug-like response. It's like if somebody shot up with heroin, you know. It takes my stress level immediately from up here and drops it, and *keeps* it down there for a while. It doesn't just come running right back up again.

. . . .

A woman's body may also secrete painkillers in response to stresses that remind her of the original events.[18] Such reminders can prompt the body to secrete painkillers equivalent to eight milligrams of morphine,[19] decreasing psychological distress. According to one theory, because an abused woman unconsciously needs the same "drug" response she experienced during the original abuse, she may seek sex with multiple strangers, find herself attracted to an abusive partner, or inflict the same abuse upon others or upon herself.[20]

It seems that the drug effect of self-injury may wane over the years. Barbara, who has been cutting herself for seventeen years, eventually realized that it no longer always brought some of the desired feelings of relief. The fact that cutting has lost its effectiveness has encouraged her to look for alternative, socially acceptable ways of living with her emotions.

Scenes from the lives of abused women who self-injure link the abusive past to their present actions:

. . . .

Elizabeth: Sometimes, depending on how bad I am, I need to go very deep. [For example] if something happened that day, like, my brother who abused me when I was fifteen, we work in the same building. And he has this habit where he won't call me by my name; he calls me Ugly. And that really affects me. And that will be what triggers it, but then when I start cutting, it's *everything* that he did. And I'll cut, and I'll know that it's deep and it's bleeding, and I'll know it's bad, but I still don't feel that everything he's done is gone. So I'll do it again. And I'll just keep going deeper, and deeper, and deeper until I have a big opening. I just keep going over it and over it and over it. And that's why I've got really bad scars that I know are never going to go away.

. . .

Rosa: I have this nasty burn on the inside of my forearm that I got last year. And I can't say it was done on purpose but it was shortly after my father came to my house and I was ironing my clothes. And the iron fell over and the edge of it caught my arm. I should have let it drop. Instead I tried to catch it and it caught my arm, so I had this long burn, and I picked on it a couple of times. Then I was really good and I stopped picking on it and I let it heal.

. . .

Karen: The vaginal cutting usually happens after my father's done something provocative to me. He'll send me something in the mail that's, you know, gross, something that is upsetting to me. He once sent me a picture of himself, with his genitals. He's done things in the past, like, he'll be sitting on the couch and if there's laundry on the couch he might put my underpants

over his face and make gestures. You know, things like that that are *obvious* —
I can't ignore the meaning in them.

. . . .

Elizabeth, Rosa, and Karen illustrate self-injury as an immediate reaction to
the perpetrators of their childhood abuse even though years have passed since
the original abuse occurred. In Rosa's case, her self-injury was probably not
quite accidental, given the context of her story and the words she uses: "I can't
say it was done on purpose but it was shortly after my father came to my
house."

Another example is Susan, a woman who considers herself "accident
prone." She does not consciously intend to harm herself, but repeatedly does
so, especially by "accidentally" burning herself while ironing. During childhood, she was repeatedly sexually molested by a schoolfriend's father. As a
person who self-injures only through relatively mild "accidents," Susan illustrates a theory: abuse has the most devastating impact when the abuser is one
of the child's caregivers.[21] When the sexual abuser is not a caregiver, the violation of trust and attachment is not as damaging, and the biological stress
system's response and the subsequent self-injury may be less severe.[22] Susan's
abuser was not a family member and Susan was already old enough to be in
school when the abuse first occurred, factors that may have protected her from
direct self-injury. Also, Susan may have been spared the feelings of worthlessness and ugliness that encourage direct self-injury and can result from repeated sexual, physical, or emotional abuse by a caregiver.

The importance of childhood attachments may be one reason that women
who self-injure often try to shield a parent from blame for past abuse. It is
painful to fully acknowledge that the object of a woman's attempts at early
attachment was her abuser. As Meredith says, "It's easier for me to believe that
I'm evil, horrible, vile and that the reason that all this stuff happened to me
was because I am that person. It's much easier for me to believe that than to
believe that the people around me did this." Women may also be reluctant to
fully place the blame on their abusers because the abuse often begins between
the ages of two and seven, a stage during which children tend to believe that
they are to blame for anything that goes wrong. Self-blame then remains with
a traumatized child into adulthood, leading a woman to feel ashamed of having been abused. Her tendency to feel guilty is even greater if she was sexually
aroused by or felt good about any aspect of the abuse, such as the personal
attention.[23] Also, her abuser may have repeatedly told her that she was "asking for it" or that the sexual abuse was a sign of love or a form of sex educa-

tion, causing shame, guilt, and confusion to torment a woman who rationally knows she was helpless and innocent:

. . . .

Edith: Of course the message the kid gets out of all this is: "I'm bad." That's the thing [my therapist and I] have been working on for so long, because there are still pieces of: "It's *my* fault; *I'm* bad; *I'm* rotten; *I* did this; *I'm* the person to blame."

. . . .

Shame and the perceived need for self-punishment or self-discipline are understandable for a person who currently feels, as Edith did during childhood, that she caused her own abuse. If the child was drugged before the abuse or told afterward that nothing had happened, she may be confused about reality and about her subsequent emotional pain. Self-injury becomes visible "proof" that her emotions are real and valid.

All women who participated in this project said that they injured themselves, sometimes or always, in response to a variety of emotions: "Whenever I feel really stressed out," "I don't know what to do with the tension inside me," "My thoughts take a plummet," "I have an overwhelming feeling of— whatever," "There's anxiety building up," "I just feel so much emotion." These emotional states reflect biological processes (altered patterns of neurons, kindling, stress hormone imbalances). Early memories of self-injury can help explain how it is that self-injury seems the only outlet for many abused women's emotions. Elizabeth first started injuring herself as a teenager. When her father, who had sexually molested her as a child, was physically violent, she would go upstairs with a frustration that would not come out and that felt like a physical presence: "it seemed like it was *stuck* here in my chest." She would bang her head against the wall or get her father's hammer from the tool shed and beat herself. This way of releasing her frustration did not feel strange to her; she thought it normal.

Peggy also gives an interesting account of her initial experiences with emotions and self-injury.

. . . .

When I was a kid, [pain] used to be the point [of self-injury]: until it started to hurt [the feeling] wouldn't decrease. I did it until it hurt; it was supposed to hurt. . . . The choice was: I can explode inside or I can do this. The choice was to live with that feeling or hurt myself, which helped it to go away. I guess it's anger, but it's more than that: it's rage. It's even more than that, it's so many things at once: "This has happened: I've tried this to make it not happen, and it still happened; I've tried this to make it not happen, and it still happened; I've tried *this*, it still happened and I'm still dealing with this." I was totally trapped. There was no way that I could change my behavior or do anything different to try and prevent the kind of abuse that I dealt with on a daily basis. So it just built up so much that it felt like my insides were literally going to explode. All this rage that had to come out somehow, and I just couldn't come up with any other way to get it all out. Were there other ways? I don't know; probably. I couldn't talk about it, none of the usual ways were available to me, so that's what I did.

. . . .

Faced with the overwhelming emotions of daily abuse and with "none of the usual ways" available to express them, what else is a child to do? If she had been older, she might have turned to alcohol or other drugs or even to binge-eating and perhaps purging to numb and control her explosive emotions. Being so young, however, she turned to the most basic means available: her own body.

Sometimes a step called dissociation, discussed in the prologue, occurs between the emotion and self-injury, especially self-cutting. A severe form of dissociation bans all emotions and sensations from consciousness and can feel like a form of death — no emotions, no sensations, and little ability to move or speak: "It's like there's somebody in there that tells me I'm going to do it"; "It's like being bound in cotton — I just can't move"; "I'm feeling like I'm not anywhere, like I'm floating up in space"; "I'm there, but I'm not connected to myself." These are descriptions of the varying degrees of dissociation experienced by some women before cutting themselves. When a woman cuts to bring herself back into her body, it is like a return to life. This is an ironic fact, given the negative connotations of a self-inflicted wound and the tendency to consider cutting self-destructive.

Each woman's act of self-injury says something, such as "I hate myself," "I'm enraged," "I can't bear feeling separate from my body," "I need help." At times, it expresses many things at once, including the underlying statement that "Right now, I cannot express myself in socially acceptable ways." In traumatized women, self-injury may also be saying that "It was never safe to speak out, cry, or shout; I couldn't even tell anyone what was happening to me. This is how I silently speak, tell, cry, and shout."

Traumatized women who injure themselves generally experience their first trauma before puberty and often in early childhood,[24] a time when all of us react to the world through our senses and actions more than through words.

As we begin to express ourselves through speech, maltreatment can impair our ability to express specific emotions verbally.[25] Sometimes the maltreatment is accompanied by prohibitions against any expression of anger or distress. If violence or threat of violence is a parent's response to problems, a child who has no other role models has no one from whom to learn how to talk to solve problems, and no one who will listen. Therefore, women who experienced trauma as children are more likely to react with physical sensations and actions than with words. The actions may be directed outwardly as aggression, toward one's own body as self-injury, or both; and they may begin in childhood, adolescence, or adulthood. Self-injury then becomes a form of communication that reveals the unspeakable. This is one explanation for self-injury as a response to childhood abuse and for abused women's problems with words. Women who self-injure often cannot express their feelings in words and say that there are no words for such feelings.

Edith and Esther used to injure their hands, wondering as they did so why they were injuring a part of their bodies impossible to conceal. Edith concluded that it was a way of saying "Look, look, do you see how much pain I'm in? *This* is how much pain I'm in." Esther realized that she was trying to let her therapist know how much she hurt inside. When she was able to tell him this and he acknowledged it, she stopped cutting her hands. Other women also say that cutting their hands is a way of saying "Help me," because they do not know how to ask in any other way or they fear that their words will be ignored.[26] Erica once cut herself in front of another person but emphasized that the situation and her reaction were unusual: her cut was in anger at the person in the room. "It was me saying to this woman: 'This is how it makes me feel.'" Usually, her self-injury is private and concealed, yet still a form of communication.

Some women cut letters or words into their skin. These have a special, personal meaning — for example, the words "bad" and "evil" can show how a woman felt about herself when she cut. One woman thought that if she spoke these thoughts rather than cut them, no one would understand.[27] Other women paint pictures or write with their blood. Barbara once wrote "Blood speaks louder than words," an opinion many women who self-injure share.

Together, therefore, the pieces of a woman's past that seem to underlie self-injury form a mosaic that includes:

1. trauma-related imbalances in the body's stress response system
2. a need to express emotions without using words
3. dissociation, sometimes to the point of having other identities

4. periodic feelings that are identical to or closely resemble those experienced during abuse that occurred years before
5. a retained sense of guilt left over from a child's sense of responsibility for her own abuse and shame about her "badness"
6. a need for visible evidence that past memories and current emotions are real and valid

With this mosaic in mind, the feelings that precipitate self-injury become clearer and self-injury becomes a comprehensible, logical release to a person living with the aftermath of childhood abuse.

Nonetheless, in addition to the links between prior abuse and self-injury, "nature" may play a role, at least for some women: an abused woman's genetic inheritance may help determine how she will react to such abuse. Any parent who sexually, physically, or emotionally abuses an offspring has profound problems of his or her own that could include a tendency toward volatile emotions. If this tendency is partly genetic and is passed on to the abused child, self-injury may sometimes be related to genetic susceptibility as well as to the experience of abuse.

A child can also learn by imitating a parent's behavior (nurture) and, perhaps, be genetically inclined toward such behavior (nature). Caroline thinks that she tended to imitate her parents' mode of anger: explode, lash out, then calm down soon afterward. Now, she is trying to imitate people whose reactions to anger are less upsetting and do not lead to lashing out or to self-injury. Jessica's daughter once cut herself, then repeatedly scratched herself when she felt overwhelmed between the ages of fourteen and twenty. Jessica does not know the exact cause of her daughter's self-injury but suspects that inheriting Jessica's "high-strung" temperament and imitating Jessica's self-cutting were two possible factors among others, such as witnessing violence at home. These factors combined would give nature and nurture shared roles in Jessica's daughter's self-injury.

Edith and Rosa each think that one of their parents (father and mother respectively) chronically self-injured. Edith and Barbara suspect that their mothers had multiple identities. Nonetheless, these patterns do not necessarily suggest that Edith or Barbara genetically "inherited" self-injury or multiple identities from their parents or that they imitated the parent's behavior. A more likely explanation is that these parents were abused as children. Supporting this view is a study showing that a parent's self-injury did not lead to her or his child's self-injury.[28] Of the mothers I interviewed, only one reported that her child self-injured. Also, self-injury occurs after abuse or neglect by adoptive parents, foster parents, or strangers, indicating that the trauma of prolonged childhood abuse is a sufficient catalyst for self-injury; neither imitation nor genetic inheritance is necessary.

A key topic in the nature versus nurture debate is the role of women's anger in self-injury. One of the unspoken emotions expressed through self-injury is something my informants usually call "anger," a term that may sometimes convey what they feel. Yet, I think that anger is often too mild a word to express the emotion that self-injuring women experience or fear to experience. Murderous rage that feels like it could swell into uncontrollable violence or lead to momentary or permanent insanity is more descriptive of the feeling that women fear and stifle through self-injury. Rage, defined as violent and uncontrolled anger,[29] often cannot be expressed through speech and can perhaps be called the boiling point of speechlessness.[30] With repeated abuse as part of one's past, this boiling point can be quickly reached. Sarah uses the term "anger" but defines it as physical manifestations: her jaw clenches, she shakes, and her vision changes, making her almost "see red." These physical sensations seem to require physical release. As an adolescent, Sarah would release them through fights. Nowadays, Sarah gets angry at herself for being angry and has to restrain herself from the urge for self-punishment through cutting. She thinks that her unreleased anger becomes an ache in her body for cutting. The physical sensations of anger evolve into physical pain that demands physical release, and all without a word spoken.

Elizabeth's experiences with "anger" are similar. As a child, she was not allowed to express anger even though her father and mother had fits of rage that they took out on their children at the slightest provocation. In self-defense, Elizabeth developed what she calls a "good-little-girl attitude": she kept everything inside and never showed anger. As the years went by, Elizabeth found that she could not express anger even in physically safe situations. Now, as an adult, feeling angry frightens Elizabeth and she fears losing control, a familiar theme among women who injure themselves. Elizabeth says that she has so much anger inside that if she tried to let part of it out, all of it would escape and her mind would "go" or she would harm someone. She finds it easier to keep her anger inside until she can discharge it through self-injury:

. . . .

I'd rather not say anything at all and keep the peace than say something and have somebody mad at me. My counselor is always saying to me, "Now, when that person said that to you, why didn't you stand up for yourself and say, 'I don't appreciate that.'" Like when my brother calls me Ugly. "Why didn't you say, 'I do not appreciate you calling me Ugly. Call me by my name.'" And I said, "Because then he would get mad at me, and then I would be upset, and then it would make things worse. It's better to say nothing at all and just keep the peace." And she said, "Yeah, but then it affects you inside in the long run." But I said, "I'm fine with that." I'm used to it. I can just go up to my room and cut, or beat myself with a hammer. It's easier that way. Because then I don't have to deal with other people's anger and with conflict and confrontation. I can be real calm about it and say, "Whatever you say," and just agree with them and go along with it and take whatever comes — and then I can go away and cut. To me, it just seems easier.

· · · · · · · · ·

Women's anger and rage repeatedly emerge as feared and disallowed emotions expressed through cutting, hitting, or burning their own bodies. The angry woman may think "I'll show you!" — referring to the person she is angry with — then secretly cut herself as her way of "showing." Or she may feel angry, then censor her anger as an emotion she should not feel. Jane's experiences are one example of anger's power. As a child, Jane was punished if she showed anger. Now a mother herself, Jane sometimes expresses her anger by yelling at her children or slamming doors. She also buries her anger so that it makes her sick with a stomachache or cramps, or secretly vents it by denying herself something, clawing her body, or cutting herself. She gets angry at someone or something, then is angry with herself for being angry "because I'm not supposed to get angry." For a long time, Jane could not tolerate the mention of anger: she would dissociate each time her therapist brought up the subject. Jane says that most of the time she still does not recognize her own anger although she can now discuss it without dissociating.

Edith calls anger "the topic of the moment." When I talked with her, she had recently begun to be angry about "everything," even things that are not important to her. She also found this thought coming up: "How *dare* you do that to me," conveying a right to be treated well and to set limits, rights impossible to demand or enforce as a child. Edith's anger coincided with an attempt to stop picking at her skin for a while, but Edith noticed the anger even somewhat prior to stopping:

· · · · · · · · ·

I finally realized what I've been doing with my picking all these years. I've always talked about being a volcano that was getting ready to erupt. And what I've been doing with the picking is making little vents in the bottom of the volcano so that it never went over. And when I stopped making vents, then the anger started to go over. So, my therapists have been asking me a lot lately, "Now, what are you really angry at?" I know the answer to that, logically, but I can't feel it emotionally yet. The answer is, I'm angry about what was done to me as a child. I know that, [but] it's not in my core, in the feeling part of me yet. So I get mad at my therapists, and I get mad at other people, and I get mad at things. . . . But clearly, for me, the payoff for not picking is letting the anger get up to the point where I can recognize it and deal with it and be *done* with it, so that it's not in there just tearing me up, and I'm tearing me up to keep from feeling.

. . . .

Festering rage is an expected response to abuse,[31] though it is usually not expressed in words, and men and women differ in their nonverbal expressions of posttraumatic rage. Research suggests that among men and women abused as children, men tend to become aggressive or violent toward others, while women are more likely to be resigned or depressed or to injure themselves or attempt suicide.[32] Even when abused women and men experience the same feelings of worthlessness, hopelessness, shame, or guilt, women are more likely to injure themselves or attempt suicide while men are more likely to act aggressively toward others.

For some women, self-injury occasionally serves the purpose of keeping them from becoming violent. They say that their anger is too dangerous to feel because it might swell into violent rage.

. . . .

Rosa: Sometimes I get really afraid of my anger. I don't like it because when my anger comes out full blown, it's rage and I want to break things and I want to hurt things. I want to hurt the person I'm angry with because that's the kind of anger that I dealt with; that's what I learned. So with my lover Joan, I told her and all my lovers that there are times when I get really angry and I just need to take a break and a walk and calm down because I get so angry I want to put my fists through somebody's face. If I can't calm myself down, then I usually end up hurting myself later because I take the anger out on me.

. . . .

Edith, too, fears even starting to be angry because her anger might build to the point of her going amok: rip the curtains off the wall and the telephone from its socket, throw over tables and chairs, and hurl objects through windows. Self-injury releases the anger before it can become rage and violence. As a child, Edith used to daydream about having one of her teachers, a six-foot-six man, restrain her rage. In her fantasy she thought about being physically, violently out of control but being "rescued" by this teacher who would hold her until she could stop. Edith's interesting fantasy turned her teacher into a living safety valve, playing the same role as her picking and cutting, and revealing her fear of violence. Edith fears this violence even though her fantasy of what she might do in rage does not include injuring people.

Three of the women I talked with have felt the urge to harm another person, and two of the three have done so. As a teenager, Sarah once during a fight bit her cousin, drawing blood, and on two occasions slapped or pushed her mother, imitating her father and showing that she could disobey her mother's orders to stay home. Karen, in a distraught state after a long hospitalization, once physically abused her daughter. Karen's self-cutting frequently results from urges to cut her husband. She once called an emergency hotline to report that she was going to slit her sleeping husband's throat, and has also threatened to cut her therapist. Yet, the part of her that resists cutting others has always pulled her back, and she hasn't cut others "yet." When I asked if cutting others was a possibility, Karen replied: "I hope it isn't."

Interestingly, Edith and Barbara allow themselves to feel their rage only through a male alter identity, a part of themselves that split off as a result of childhood abuse. Edith has an alter identity called George who has shown his/her rage by smashing a tennis racket and punching the wall so hard he broke the bracelet Edith was wearing. Edith remembers that once during a hospitalization she found herself barricaded in a corner by several of the staff who were holding her on both sides. She did not know why she was being held until the staff explained: "George was out." George might once have caused Edith's arrest if a police officer had happened by when s/he was throwing over a picnic table and picking up and throwing the benches in a small park behind a cinema. Edith had just seen a film showing injustice and violence, situations so much a part of her childhood experiences. As she was throwing the furniture, she noticed glass on the ground and thought, "I'm going to cut"—a clear sign of wanting to be violent and cut in response to rage.

Barbara says that she generally doesn't express anger well but cuts instead, sometimes deeply, because her anger makes her want to destroy or carve into something. Barbara is afraid of anger because she feels the potential for violence: "I've had a lot of violence done to me and I was always determined to never do violence to anyone else. I have kept to that." She feels that anger makes her evil, mean, hurtful, and sadistic like her abusers, and this equation makes her angry at herself, sometimes leading to severe cutting. Barbara has punched holes in walls before but manages to control herself during impulses to hurt someone: "I would feel so bad if I lost it on anyone." If anger surfaces, Barbara switches to a male alter called Slugger who is "very bad," sadistic, and whose role is to feel Barbara's anger. Because of this anger, Slugger also cuts

Barbara severely, once almost to the bone. Barbara had a revealing experience when her therapist encouraged her to feel her anger without escaping into Slugger:

. . . .

My therapist hates me to leave a session mad. I do get into a rage sometimes, and sometimes [my therapist] won't let me switch. Like I switched, [so] I said, "*I'm* not angry" because I think it's not me; I think it's Slugger's anger. And she's like, "No, repeat after me: *I'm* angry" and I go, "You're angry." I give her a hard time. And she finally makes me try to see that if Slugger's angry, I'm angry: to try to identify with my anger. And one day she really got me to. . . . I just felt like I could feel rage in *me*, not just me being Slugger, but *I* could feel it. I couldn't deal with it. She was trying to make me write a contract for safety, and I broke the pen in half. And she goes, "Here, scribble on this piece of paper." She had a clipboard under it, and I scribbled so hard on the piece of paper it dug straight through the clipboard. And I ripped my clothes! I was wearing a heavy wool coat and I ripped the coat in half and bit the buttons off it, and I was wanting to break glass in the office and to just leave. I said, "I have to leave," and she said, "I can't let you leave like this," and I just wanted to go crash my car into things, or break everything—I wanted to cut, too, I mainly wanted to cut. I kept looking around her office for something sharp. I ended up calming down and I didn't cut, but I felt like, because of the anger, that's what I wanted to do.

. . . .

Edith/George and Barbara/Slugger seem to illustrate the social norm that violence toward things or people is largely a male prerogative. Violence by men is also socially more acceptable than is self-injury: our eyes are accustomed to seeing it, our ears to hearing it. Some men earn high wages for hitting each other in public (boxing), or by playing aggressive, injury-prone sports such as football. Such sports also provide abused boys and men with socially acceptable ways to be injured and to hurt others.[33] Peggy illustrates this social acceptance of violence when she says that she feels less self-conscious if her son happens to see her kick or punch the wall than when he catches her banging her head. Lashing out to hurt something or someone else is "normal"; injuring herself is not.

Self-injuring women's fantasies of revenge on their abusers usually reveal that their rage is socially harmless. Edith used to plan to kill her father and would say that the only thing that prevented her was the thought of spending the rest of her life in prison. She would fantasize about going with a gun in her hand to her father's house while he was sleeping. Yet, Edith finally realized that even in her imagination, she does not shoot her father in bed but instead makes a noise that awakens him so that he comes out of the bedroom and is terrified by the sight of her standing before him with a gun in her hand. The point is to terrify her father by threatening violence, not to carry it out.

Similarly, the story that Erica told herself from her eighth year did not allow violent retaliation against her abusive mother. Instead, every night before she went to bed, Erica would tell herself the elaborate fiction that the abusive adults in her house were impostors, not her real parents. In Erica's fantasy, the loving parents of a friend discover that Erica's parents are abusive impostors and try to protect Erica. In her thirties, Erica added a scene in which the impostors meet gory, violent deaths. Erica told herself this additional story for ten years every night before she went to bed. In this ingenious way, Erica constructed a story in which her plight was recognized, she was rescued, and her abuser was punished with violence, all without Erica accusing or destroying her mother even in Erica's imagination. Erica's restraint may have been due not only to her gender but to the fact that her abuser was a parent. As Mary confirms, "It's a lot harder to have [revenge] thoughts about your parents. It's easier to have those thoughts about . . . strangers that hurt you."

Yet, some women do have "those thoughts." Esther is one who, in her imagination, uses violence to avenge herself against the father who abused her physically and sexually. She describes her fantasies:

. . . .

I'm an eight-year-old girl and my father is on top of me forcing himself on me sexually. I have a knife underneath the pillow and I pull it out and stab him in the back. He dies and I cut him up into little pieces. That's one. Another one: I'm a much younger child, three or four years old, and instead of lying still on the stone table, she sits up and takes the knife away from the man who owns it and cuts down his face.

. . . .

Esther considers these fantasies positive because they show her as an empowered little girl rather than "lying still" as she was so often compelled to do. Even though fantasy shows her murdering and chopping into pieces her father who repeatedly raped her, in reality Esther cannot bear the sight of someone else's blood and refuses to watch the "slasher" movies her husband loves. Also, most of the people in Esther's revenge fantasies are dead, which possibly explains why she allows her imagination to play with the idea of gory violence toward her late father.

Edith stops short of actual violence when imagining revenge on her father, while Erica and Esther seem to strictly control the circumstances under which their imaginations are allowed full play. Even in these three women's minds, violence is threatened but not committed, or is reserved for those who are not a parent or for a parent safely dead.

Male violence, so much a part of everyday life, can sometimes be explained as childhood abuse's effects: a highly excitable stress-response system, low self-esteem, and the need to use action rather than words. Like self-injury, aggression toward others is known to be an abused person's attempt to regulate emotions.[34] Childhood abuse and/or neglect can lead a person to become impulsive, irritable, hypervigilant, and unusually distrustful and can diminish a person's judgement, empathy, and verbal abilities—all characteristics that can make men prone to violence. In every culture, men commit the vast majority of crimes[35] and men abused or neglected as children become violent criminals more often than unabused men or abused or unabused women.[36] Yet, when violent men are prevented from violence because they are hospitalized or imprisoned, they can become depressed, self-injurious, and suicidal.[37] In other words, they tend to feel and behave like abused women. Some invisible "hospital" or "prison" seems to keep most abused women from becoming public menaces like some of their male counterparts. Perhaps aggressiveness is influenced by androgen and testosterone[38]—two hormones higher in men than in women—as well as by social expectations about how boys and girls should behave. Thus, nature and nurture may combine to encourage abused women to express their speechless rage through their own bodies.

3 *Meredith Tells Her Story*

In Her Twenty-sixth Year of Life and Eleventh Year of Self-Injury

SOME OF what I hear myself say to you in response to your questions leaves me a little shaken because it makes it all very real to me. And part of the reason why I'm doing this [interview] is because it's making it real to me; it's not something that I can deny. Some of the answers that I have for you *are* disturbing, and it is disturbing to me to hear myself say that I think I should be treated this way. I wouldn't say that it's a negative thing, though. I think that it's illustrating to me that I do want my life to be different and I do want to be able to function differently in the world than I've been functioning for the last twenty-six years, and in a less painful way.

I attribute [self-injury's] existence to the trauma in my early life. . . . [My mother] hit us a lot; she would pick things up and hit us with things [and also slapped and pinched us]. She would say things like, "How can you stand to look at yourself? You're so gross." She would stand me in the mirror and stand behind me and say, "Look at yourself. Look how ugly you are." [Also], I remember this one period of time when my father was having an affair. I was probably eleven or twelve and my brother was six or seven. For months she took us out until 4 A.M. on a regular basis to stalk my father's lover.

[Concerning my father] there's so much I don't remember. I know that my brother and I were forced to be physically intimate with one another and that there was some taking of pornographic pictures of me and I'm not sure about my brother. That's really all I remember right now. I'd say I started to remember on the day my father died. [Before that] I had been hospitalized and had some psych testing and I had all these signs and symptoms, and some people told me that they suspected. And I was like, "No way! I don't know what you're talking about." Then about a year and a half later my father died. On the night that he died, I had this dream about it, and I woke up, and I knew. It was bizarre because here was my whole family and they were devastated because my father died very unexpectedly at forty-eight. And I wasn't devastated at all because of this newfound information. [Now] I have dreams about it all the time; but not dreams that give me any more of the pieces. It's more like even though the dream isn't about it, the latent content is, and I'll wake up and be upset.

[Now], I don't really have relationships with men because they scare me to death. . . . I'm very distrustful of them. If it's in a social situation where it's a friend of a friend, I can talk to them or if it's my friend's boyfriend or husband, that's okay. But for me to talk to men that I don't know, I can't do that. I'm very conscious of myself and how ugly I am, or how ugly I feel, and that gets in the way. I'm very distrustful and very frightened of them. I don't understand them; they scare me. I think that they are all horrible people and shouldn't be trusted. My therapist and I talk about this a lot, and how not all men are like that. And [it] blows my mind . . . that it actually could be nice to be touched in that way by someone you care about or that you could tell your husband what your feelings were and what happened when you were younger. There are people in my life who are married who do share [abusive pasts] with their husbands and say that having sex with their husbands is a wonderful thing. That's mind-blowing to me; I just don't get that.

[It's possible for me to have sex with some men] because my feeling for them is one of disdain and repulsion. I don't know if this is going to make any sense — it's a power thing: it allows me to feel like I'm controlling them, and that, to me, makes them weak. If they're weak, then they're not frightening to me because if I'm more powerful than they are, they can't hurt me.

I'm just going to say it and not even worry about what you think about it: I have never had sex with anyone that I care about. To me that is the most vulgar thing someone could ever do and I don't understand how or why people could do that with people they care about. I can't imagine doing that, so I [have sex with people I don't care about] because, other than cutting, it is the area in my life that gives the feeling of having power; having power over the person I'm doing it with, or I guess, doing it *to* would be the more accurate description. . . . I think I do it because maybe I'm hoping that this time it will be different and nice, which it never has been. [Also], I think that it gives me a tremendous feeling of power because I can make him want me; I can make him feel really good; and I have total control because if I stop, then he doesn't have that any more and he'll ask me for more.

Physically, I can feel [the sex], but it doesn't feel good, it feels pretty horrible actually. Emotionally, at the time, the only thing I can feel is this overwhelming sense of power and that blocks all the other feelings. But after it's done, I feel horrible. I always have a hard time afterwards: I feel like a whore and a slut.

One thing that makes me want to cut myself a lot is — this is going to sound paradoxical! — feeling like I want other people to care about me. . . .

It's absolutely intolerable to me that I want other people to care about me. Two women I was hospitalized with [once] told me that they cared about me, and they gave me a gift. I couldn't handle it. I don't fully understand [why it was intolerable for me, but] . . . I think part of it is, on some level, it feels like they shouldn't be the people caring about me; it should have been my parents. And so, the difficulty isn't with getting it, it's with having had to wait so long to get it. I think [another] part is that I absolutely do not understand how anyone could care about me, or like me, or want to be friends with me, or spend time with me, or enjoy my company—or anything. I think that's connected to feeling [that] I don't deserve for them to care about me: I'm this horrible, evil, vile, disgusting, twisted, warped individual and it's arrogant to want people to care about me.

I have worked with [my therapist] for over three years. I just looked at her for the first time about four weeks ago. In our sessions before, I had never looked at her: I looked at her feet or I looked at the door, I looked at the wall, I looked at the rug; I never looked at her. I would look at her [when] she had to get up to walk over to her desk to get something. But I never looked at her while we were talking, and I never looked at her in the face. I didn't even know what she looked like. She used to question me about it sometimes and we talked about it. My concern was always that she was going to think that I was being dishonest with her because when people don't look at you when they're talking to you, that can be a sign that they're not being truthful. But we talked about it and she understands it. I'm telling you this [because it] is connected to my not feeling like I deserve [to have] other people care about me. Part of why I was not able to look at her is because I kind of felt like, "Who am I to look at her? I don't have that right; I don't deserve that; that [would be] an insult to her." That's part of it, [and the other part is] my being so horribly, painfully ashamed of what I'm telling her, and of myself.

I have come to understand [the cutting] as a way for me to try to have some control in my life because when I was younger, there wasn't anything in my control; that was the only thing I had. I think when it first started it didn't have as many functions and purposes as it does now [and] . . . I didn't do it as frequently, as deeply, and as many times in one episode as I do it now.

I cut myself in places that can be easily covered by clothing and I don't wear clothing that would reveal them. When I was younger I used to do it . . . on the insides of the bottom of my legs. [Also], my left forearm is pretty scarred up, but those scars are just little ones, so they can be explained away. I have some that cannot be explained away on my shoulders, so I don't wear sleeveless things . . . and some on my chest, but they can be covered by clothes. My legs can be covered up easily. . . . [So] if I have gaping wounds on my upper thigh, I put on a pair of pants and no one knows. There are places that I want to do it: my lower forearm and my face, but I don't for those reasons. [I think I want to cut on those places] because I can see the forearm [and] I would be able to look. And the face, because I want to disfigure myself—this is just a guess—so that the outside can match my perceived inside. Because if I did it to my face, [that] would be a reflection of what's inside. Then everyone else would be able to know that I'm this disfigured individual. When people look at you, the first thing they see is your face, so they would be looking at what's inside [and] know how horrible it was. Then I wouldn't be able to fool people and I wouldn't be so deceitful to them. They would look at me and they would know. The way that I look at it is, no one knows how evil I am, and if they could see it, then they would know the real truth.

It serves a lot of functions in my life. I use it as a way to punish myself, I use it as a way to medicate myself, I use it for the tension release when things get too strong or too built up. When I first started doing it about eleven years ago, the cuts were just scratching. They were in places that were visible, like on my wrists [on the inside]. At that time I don't really know what the motivation was, but attention was part of it. It was kind of shocking to people. I'm not quite sure why it started; not sure what was going through my mind. I didn't do it for a while, and when I started again I did it in places that people couldn't see. And then the more I did it, the more secret it became. . . .

I call it an addiction because I absolutely can't stop doing it and I love to do it and it gives me a high like nothing else does: no chemical I've ever ingested; like nothing I've ever ingested. [By high I mean] a feeling of euphoria, like a total rush through my body. While I'm doing it, and sometimes before, my heart is racing, my body is tingling. When I'm done, after this big huge buildup, then there's an overwhelming feeling of calmness, an overwhelming sense of peace. And the more I do it the more I have to do it to produce the same effects. I think about it all the time, I want to do it all the time, there's not a day that goes by that I don't want to do it—never, never. . . . When things are harder I want to do it more, and it's harder for me not to do it. If it's just a regular day, something silly will happen, and I'll want to do it but it will just be, "Oh, I want to" and that's it. Other times it will be, "I need to, I need to, I have to." And those are the days I have to work hard not to.

I use these things called "utility blades"; they're big, thick razor blades. I go into the bathroom and I take everything I'm going to need, like a washcloth and a towel and something to put on it afterwards if it bleeds. Then I sit in the tub and I start cutting myself. When I start, they're shallow, small cuts, and by the time I'm done, they're big and deep. Then I sit there and I let myself bleed for a while, for a long while, usually half an hour. Then I take a shower to get all the blood off me and because the warm water makes the blood look like more [and] makes my legs bleed longer. When I feel like I'm done and don't need to do it anymore, then I turn the shower off, dry off, and take a wet washcloth and put pressure on the cuts on my legs until they stop bleeding. Then I go and watch television or something and I have to sit on towels because my legs continue to bleed and I don't want to get it on the furniture. [While watching] television, I always put my hands on [the cuts] and feel them and look at them. I'm *obsessed* with looking at them for the next couple of days. It gives me a rush. Even if I can't see them, I can put my hand on my leg where they are and I can feel them. Even if I'm wearing a skirt, I can feel them under the skirt, know that they're there — *Wow*, that was hard for me to say! This is making it very real to me; hearing myself say all this is giving me a clearer sense of how real this stuff is and, like, this wouldn't exist if my life wasn't horrible. It kind of gives more credence to the things that I think happened when I was younger — just hard.

I live with an incredible amount of pain [but] none of it comes from what I do to myself. I feel [the cutting] but it doesn't hurt. . . . It's kind of like I can feel it cutting my skin and I can feel that it's happening, but it's not painful to me. . . .

I think when [my therapist] and I talk about things that are really, really hard, that sometimes makes me want to cut more. Sometimes it's not necessarily that *that* in itself makes me want to cut. It might be more like we talk about something really hard, I have a lot of feelings, I'm overwhelmed, I come home and I can't find my keys, and I want to cut myself. But it's not really because I can't find my keys.

[Sometimes I do it for relief because things are] mixed up. It's like everything inside is churning and tumbling around all over the place: I can't sit still, my mind is going a million miles an hour, I'm having all these feelings, and I'm overwhelmed. . . . That's the only way I know how to calm things down. [At other times] I have this governing belief that I need to be punished for being the kind of person I'm being; doing the things I've done — just, I need to be punished: I can't really explain the why behind it. Sometimes it's as simple as I'll be doing the dishes and drop a plastic cup onto the floor. And I'll be like, "You're so stupid; you're such an idiot; you should cut yourself; blah, blah, blah." Sometimes it's a little bit more sophisticated than that. It's like my thinking about the type of person that I am and needing to be punished for that. I think that I'm manipulative, dishonest, evil, and vile, vile.

[By manipulative I mean] I think I've made all this up, none of it exists, like it's all a big game, I'm just doing it for attention, none of this is true, the abuse didn't happen. I think the other word for that is denial. . . .

It isn't the cut necessarily that is important to me, it is seeing my blood. . . . That's why I don't like to burn myself: there's no blood. The cut is important but only in terms of how deep it is and how much it bleeds. I guess [bleeding] is like purging to me, it's very cleansing in some sort of way. Let me think of how to say this—I know if the injury is severe enough [by] whether it bleeds and how much it bleeds. The more blood there is, the better I've cut myself. And I don't fully understand that, but I think part of it is a self-punishment thing, and if I'm bleeding, and bleeding a lot, then the injury was severe enough so it means that I punished myself. If I had cut myself and it didn't bleed, that wouldn't mean anything to me: it wouldn't have been punishment enough. Does that make sense to you? [But I don't always cut with self-punishment in mind], that's why I say that I don't fully understand it. But that's part of it. And also—I'm kind of hesitant to say this because it's really warped—but one of the things that gives me the biggest high when I'm doing it is after I've cut myself, I stand up and the blood runs down my legs and I can feel the cool blood running against my warm skin. I get really high off of that. And seeing the blood against the white towel or against the white porcelain of the tub: it's very shocking—a big contrast between those two things. And that also gives me a sense of being high: my heart's racing and I lose my breath—it's a feeling better than any drug I've ever done.

I remember one time when I was in the hospital a couple of years ago, I cut myself a lot and very, very deep. . . . I bled for three days, and that made me so high; that gave me the best feeling; that was close to the ultimate. . . . [A] couple of the women on the unit and I put in a pass together to go out to dinner. And while we were out to dinner, my legs started bleeding, and I looked down and there was blood on my coat. And that was—I don't know, like I'm starting to get high just talking about this—that was close to the ultimate for me. I remember being at the dining hall and my legs were starting to bleed, and I had to take a towel and wrap it around my legs. One of the people who work there had to help me do it because my legs were bleeding a lot. I didn't like the part about her helping me do it; I didn't like someone else seeing what I had done because to me that kind of speaks to how twisted I am, and I don't like to let other people see that. But, knowing that the injury that I had caused must have been pretty serious in order for my legs to be bleeding three days later, *that* part got me really high.

[I always cut at least fifty times each episode] because that seems to me to be severe enough. If it was just ten or twelve, it feels to me like it would be a waste of time. [Also], when I cut, if it's not deep enough to leave a scar, it's not worthwhile. I'm not really sure what that's about. . . . When I'm cutting myself, I want to be permanently scarring myself. That's another one of the goals, along with making myself bleed. . . . I don't really know how to say this — it's kind of like taking a look at what I've done to myself. And also, it's a very secretive thing and this secrecy gives me a sense of power. I can sit with my friends and I can feel on my legs through my [clothes] all the cuts, and I can be doing that right when I'm with them, and they have no idea. That gives me a tremendous sense of power.

Aside from cutting my face, the ultimate goal to me would be to cut a vein because then I would bleed a lot. And part of it is that cutting a vein or artery would be pretty serious. And, I don't mean serious in terms of requiring medical attention, because I doubt that I would go unless I was bleeding profusely for an extended period of time. But *I* would know that it was serious enough, or harsh enough, I guess, is the word. . . . And I've tried very hard to do that and I never seem to quite be able to do it.

Sometimes I'll be out in public and I'll notice the veins in people's hands, and . . . it brings up some really intense feelings for me. In that situation, the intensity with which I want to cut [is] very strong and kind of overwhelming. [I have never had the urge to cut someone else, it's just that others' veins bring up the urge for me to cut myself.] . . . I remember when I was in the hospital a few years ago — one of the women who did the psychodrama group, the vein on the back of her hands was very prominent and it stuck out. It used to freak me out because all I could think was, "God! I wish my hands were like that so that I could cut my vein" — like, it would really bother me. And on other people I'll notice how close their veins are to their skin, or when I'm meeting new people, one of the first things I'll do is look at their forearms to see if they have any cuts on their forearms — it's kind of disturbing me talking about it.

I just want to make one comment related to this: I would never, ever be as violent with someone else as I am with myself. I would never, ever be violent with anyone in any way. It's *completely* out of character. I'm very kind, caring, and considerate to other people; I'm as compassionate as I know how to be; I'm as generous and giving as I know how to be. I would never ever treat someone else the way that I treat myself. I just need to make that clear.

There was another part that I wanted to talk about briefly — and I don't know if other women have this as part of their self-injury — but the part that's most disturbing to me isn't necessarily the actual physical wound, it's more the images I see in my head when I'm *not* cutting myself. I have intrusive images of absolutely horrific scenes. In my head I see myself do things to myself that aren't even physically possible. I remember one time I was sitting in group [therapy] and all I could see was myself slitting my throat, wearing a white shirt, and the blood running and soaking the white shirt. I've seen myself stab things into my eyes [or] plunge butcher knives into my chest and cut my chest open. Slitting my throat is a big one; cutting off my limbs is something else I've seen a lot. It gets pretty graphic. Cutting my face, that's one that I see a lot because . . . the ultimate of what I could do to myself would be to scar my face. I don't allow myself to do that because I know that when it's done, I [would] wish that I hadn't, and I don't want to carry scars around on my face for the rest of my life. So I don't allow myself to, but that would be the ultimate to me. . . . Another thing is, when I have intrusive images that are not in my control, I'll see myself cut myself so deeply that there's lots of blood and it gets really gory. It's not anything that I would ever be able to actually do.

[Intrusive images like those make me feel] crazy, crazy. That was the biggest thing that led to my last hospitalization. I *was* cutting myself, but the main reason I went to the hospital [was] because I could not stop having these intrusive images every time I looked at something or someone. For a day and a half nonstop, *nonstop* — it was horrible. [They don't give me a high or any kind of pleasurable feeling at all.] It's very, very disturbing to me; it can leave me very shaken. . . .

Those images that I just described to you are involuntary. There are times when I have voluntary images in my head. I do it on purpose because I can produce the physiological reaction that I have to cutting without cutting, by just visualizing it in my head. [In those cases the images are based on what I actually do.] . . .

[Self-injury] very much affects the way I view myself. I think it's a very poor reflection of my character because it's kind of a bizarre, whacked-out thing to do. And if I was normal and sane and wasn't such a freak, I wouldn't do it. It makes me feel very bizarre — very much separate from other people. And I don't want to create the illusion that I want to be normal, because "normal" to me sounds really boring. But, I would like to be a little less abnormal. [Less abnormal] would mean that I could spend my time and energy and efforts worrying about normal things like a job offer, job interviews, and buying a new couch, you know, quote-unquote "normal" worries, not things like "I can't do the dishes because I can't pick up the glass, because if I pick it up I'll cut myself." That just seems to be a little extreme.

I think that one of the biggest things [self-injury] does in my life is it makes me different and separate from other people. My time and my energies are focused on trying to keep myself safe as opposed to normal everyday tasks and concerns. And when I have to put so much of my time and energy into not cutting myself there's not a lot of time and energy left over for other things. I'm different than other people. Other people when they get dressed in the morning don't have to worry about dressing so that they cover up their scars, or they don't have to worry about what might happen if they start to bleed and ruin their clothes. It's not an issue for them.

I have good relationships with my friends. They don't know that I do this. One of my friends knows and we talk about it. . . . She and I used to be really close and I felt like by not sharing this with her, I was keeping part of myself from her and being dishonest with her. And I thought that she could handle it, not freak out, not be like "Oh my god, you do *what?*" I didn't feel like she would look at me differently. It's a pretty disturbing thing and some people can't handle it; some people it freaks out. She's fine with it. She doesn't like it, and she wishes that I wouldn't do it, but she understands. She dealt with bulimia for a while, and I see those two behaviors as being very similar. I think that the motivation and the feelings underneath it and the feelings that it produces in the body are similar — and the compulsion to do it and the obsessive thinking about it and the secrecy are similar. She's an incredible person and I had shared a lot of my story with her and she had been okay with all that I had shared, and I felt like I was being dishonest by not telling. That's what I feel a lot in my relationships with people: there's a whole big huge part of my world that no one even knows exists. It makes me feel dishonest and deceitful. If I'm friends with them, how can I not tell them this big part of my life? Some of my friends don't even know I'm in therapy at all. They wouldn't believe you if you told them; they would think that that was a joke! And therapy's so much a part of my life. I think that [if they knew I cut myself] they would look at me much differently and that they would think that I had a lot of problems, wasn't very stable, and was just really sick.

I have told two other people, so they know, but we've never talked about it really. One day, before I was going into the hospital, I was a complete mess: I was depressed, I wanted to die, I was cutting myself a lot, I was freaking out, I was disorganized. And my roommate called them to come over. They came over and I told them. So they know that it exists, but that's all. And they aren't really people that I have very much contact with. I care for them, we're close friends, but I don't see them very much. And then there are people who know bits and pieces of it. [So I feel it's alright to tell them lots of other things but] definitely not this because it's pretty bizarre, it's pretty shocking. I feel horrible about it, I hate the fact that I do it, I have some strong beliefs about what it means in terms of what I am as a person, and I'm not ready to share that with other people for fear that they will think the same thing: that I'm twisted and disturbed, and horrible, evil, vile.

I don't generally have a problem with [going to social events] because most of the scars are in places that can be covered up, and [visible ones] are small enough so that I can explain them away. I wouldn't go to a pool party because I wouldn't be able to wear a bathing suit: my upper thighs are pretty horribly scarred. There are other reasons that I wouldn't do it as well: I would be much too self-conscious of my body because of how I look and how I would look in a bathing suit.

[If I went swimming, the worst thing that could happen is] . . . that everyone would be able to see the scars on my legs — and they are not scars that I could explain away. Someone could comment about them and say, "What did you do to your legs?" or "What happened?" and then I would be put in a position to have to respond and any response that I would give other than the truth they wouldn't believe because my legs are so scarred up. [For explainable scars] I say that when I was younger, I was out in the woods and I fell or [that] I cut myself with a piece of glass. I take things that really did happen but didn't produce scars and I use that. Or I'll say, "The cat scratched me really bad one time" or "I was a real tomboy when I was a kid"— stuff like that.

I work on the substance abuse unit in a residential treatment facility for emotionally disturbed adolescent girls. [I see girls who self-injure and] I think that [my self-injury] gives me a more intimate understanding of what's going on. I have a different reaction than most people. I'm not so quick to label it as "Oh, she's just doing it for attention." I understand it; I *live* it every day. [Others are quick to label it but] I wouldn't so much say other people on the unit that I work on, but in other units. We have a lot of in-service and a lot of training, and that issue gets brought up sometimes, and people have some not nice things to say. . . .

Also how *I* feel when we're talking about it and people say things like "Oh, she's just doing it for attention" or "Oh, that's so gross" or stuff like that. A lot of times what I hear in people's voices is amazement, saying things like "How can she not *feel* that?" absolutely amazed. It's difficult for me; it adds to the stigma; it makes me feel more separate and more different from other people. Sometimes listening to their comments gives me more evidence of just what a freak I am.

I have a really good relationship with all the people I work with. They see me a lot different than I see me. With [one] exception, they're work relationships: I don't have contact with them outside of work. [The exception] . . . is the therapist for the kids on the unit that I work with. . . . One day I was at work and she said to me, "Are you okay? Are you okay? Why don't you come up to my office." So I went up to her office and we started talking. I didn't tell her then. We've talked a lot since then, and I told her one day. She's okay with it — again, she doesn't like that I do it; she wishes I didn't, but she didn't judge me and she's been wonderful. She didn't really say or do anything; she just sat there and continued to listen to me. That's fine. She's very kind, and caring, and gentle.

Oh my God! I don't think that [other employers or colleagues] would know what to do [if they knew] because it would be so much in contrast to how they know me. . . . And this goes back to the parts inside of me. I exist in pieces, I exist in parts. There's a very definite part of me that goes to work and that part is not the part of me that cuts. Since that's how the people I work with know me, I think that if someone told them that I [cut myself] they wouldn't believe it. One of the women I work with just started in May. And she told me that the first couple of days she worked with me, she was intimidated by me. I don't see myself like that at all. And I said, "What was intimidating about me; what did I do?" And she kept saying, "You're so composed, you're so composed." And I think that's the biggest joke ever! But that's how people at work see me: as ultra-competent, ultra-articulate, ultra-intelligent, ultra-organized. This is what she said to me: "You're always doing your job, you're always doing exactly what you need to be doing, you always know exactly what needs to be done, and you always do it exactly right." The people I work with, that is their perception of me. *Nothing* could be further from the truth. So, it's like, it wouldn't fit with what they know of me, it wouldn't fit.

[The part of me that goes to work is not the part that's talking to you now.] Actually, I don't know where that part's been and I really need for her to come back because that's also the part of me that does my schoolwork and I haven't opened a book in a month! So I need for that part to come back here. I work twenty to twenty-five hours a week at my job; I work twenty hours a week at my internship and my classes. I think the part of me that would regularly do that is on strike or something because she hasn't been going to my job [or] my internship and she certainly hasn't been doing my schoolwork. And I think that's related to — I'm getting depressed, and when I'm depressed, I don't have those abilities because my mind is so scattered. I plan on getting on some antidepressants in a very short time because it's very hard for me to pay attention to my schoolwork when all I can think of is that I want to die.

[When I go to work and that part of me is not there,] I think that I'm not as on top of things: I'm a lot less organized and less in touch with what's going on around me. I don't think it's been as noticeable to other people as it is to me because I'm only there twenty hours a week now and generally it's on the weekends, so there's not a whole lot going on. [I never have trouble remembering what happened at work.] I'm fully aware.

[If I feel the need to self-injure at work] I'll . . . make a phone call; sometimes I'll just take time by myself. There have been times in the two years that I've been at work and I've wanted to, but generally that doesn't happen, because I'm in the way of functioning at work and when I'm functioning in that way, cutting isn't really something that's part of that part of me. . . . But when that part of me doesn't go to work, that's when I have problems with it.

I'm able to keep all of my lives separate from one another. Like, my therapy life is very separate from my "regular" life, which is very separate from my work life, which is very separate from how I am at my internship, which is different from how I am at school. . . . The people that are in my work life are only in my life in that way; the people that I know through therapy are only in my life in that way; the people in my regular life don't know about my therapy life generally. And the ways that I am at those different places is very different. I would say the way that I am when I'm talking with you is a combination of how I am at work and how I am in my regular life, and a little bit of how I am in my therapy life because we're talking about that kind of stuff. But I'm not really having any feelings while we talk, and it's the part of me that goes to work and school; it functions on a very intellectual level. If I were talking with my therapist about the questions that you're asking me, it would be very difficult for me because there would be a lot of feelings. But I'm functioning in a different way right now; I'm functioning on an intellectual level, so I'm responding to you on an intellectual level and not a feeling level. . . . This is also how I am when I go to work.

I used to go to group therapy three times a week. And when I went there I very much functioned from an intellectual level. As a matter of fact, one of the other members yelled at me and said, "Don't you have feelings, Meredith? Don't you have *feelings*?" Because, this part of me doesn't have feelings, that's why I'm able to talk with you as calmly as I'm able to right now.

Everything that exists inside me exists alongside its opposite. It proves for a very confusing existence. . . . For me, it's more troublesome. For other people, they just don't get it; they think it's funny and [that] I'm strange and very original. They're used to me. They just think that I'm a weirdo; that I'm kind of out there. Someone told me once that I lived the most unique lifestyle of anyone he knows. I take that as a compliment. My friends tell me all the time that I'm a freak — they don't mean "freak" the way I mean "freak." They mean it as a compliment: that I'm very out there and do my own thing and don't care what people think. They think it's funny and in a lot of ways, I think it's funny, too. But in a lot of ways it's also very confusing and it's hard. There are times when I hear voices inside my head and I have endless, tedious, grueling debates with myself all the time. . . .

I hate [getting medical care] because I don't like strange people putting their hands on my body [and] because the possibility exists that they'll see my scars and ask questions. . . . [But] I have a very bizarre illness and no one seems to be able to diagnose it. So, I have had to go through a tremendous amount of testing, and sometimes the scars on my legs are visible. That makes me really uncomfortable. I don't have any idea [what the doctors think].

I went to a new doctor three months ago because I needed an antidepressant. We started talking about it and she found out that I cut. Her general message was that I'm a very twisted individual, I have a serious disorder that borders on schizophrenia, and I am in need of serious and intense help. Even though she said all that stuff I liked her because I respect people who say what's on their mind. Also, she has expertise in the area that my illness falls, so I went back to her. But I let her know that there were some things we needed to straighten out. I said, "I don't suffer from a departure from reality. If anything, I'm too intimately acquainted with it, and that's why I cut myself." I just clarified some misconceptions and assumptions that she had made and I let her know up front that I wasn't very happy with what she had said to me. Then she said, "Why do you think you do it?" And I said, "Do you really want the answer to that question?" And she said, "Yes." So I told her that I have come to understand my cutting as an attempt to gain some control in an absolutely out-of-control environment and that it is a sane response to an insane environment. And she asked me what I meant by that and I told her about my mother and my father. And we talked about it for a minute. And she said, "Well, this is where I stand: I will stay out of your personal life, I won't meddle in that. I will try to [take care of your illness] and that's where our work will be focused." And that's fine with me.

I also hate going to the dentist and I can't even remember the last time I went. [I hate it] because I don't like — God, this is so *Freudian* — because I don't like having people put things in my mouth. . . . Like going to the gynecologist: I can't do that either for the same reasons. And a couple of years ago I had endometriosis and I was in unbearable pain for months and months. Finally, I had to go, and it was really horrible. The nurse was wonderful, but . . . the doctor was less patient with me. Right before she started examining me I started having body memories and my body got really tense. It's kind of like my body recoils, like someone startling me and what my response would be if someone had just come up behind me and scared me — a pulling back and a flinching. Emotionally, I guess fear is what comes to mind. She wasn't very pleased. But then I was able to relax myself and the exam was over in two minutes. . . . I think the nurse was really great because she had said, "Do you have any questions or is there anything that you need to say to me?" I said, "I just want you to know that you probably see fifty people a day and this is completely normal to them, but it's not completely normal to me; it's very traumatic to me." And she asked me why and I just said, "I have had some experiences in the past where people have done things to me that I didn't want done to me." She was really great about it. She said, "Is there anything else you need to ask or you need me to tell the doctor?" I said, "I have a lot of scarring on my body and I would prefer not to be questioned about it." So, no one asked me about it. . . .

I had stopped last May, and then last week I started cutting myself again, so I hadn't been doing it for about ten months. About a month ago some really difficult stuff happened and I shut down because it was too overwhelming. I wasn't able to talk to anyone because all I knew was that something was not okay but I didn't know why it was not okay and I didn't know how to talk about it. I had remembered that part of what was included in my earlier years of abuse was that there had been some pictures that were taken, and I went home to look for them to see if I could find them.

So I went home and found a couple of them and brought them to therapy with me. We had been talking about that, and I had been having a lot of body memories: physical sensations related to the earlier abuse that happen when I talk about it. Are you sure you want me to be specific? — Oh God, I can't believe I'm saying this — Sometimes when I talk about it . . . part of what happens to my body is muscle contractions in my vagina, like my body's preparing to have sex. So, it's kind of like I'm having an orgasm, although it's not pleasurable; it's very distressing. Somehow, those things have been linked, and that's what happens. And it's triggered by talking about these kinds of things. It's also triggered when people are really nice to me and very gentle with me. That was kind of what was happening right before I shut down.

[I remember pictures that were more distressing], and I did not find those. That in itself was very distressing to me. Does that make sense? They are the ones that are most bothersome to me, and I am unable to locate them. So, where are they? and who has them? and why? and what are they doing with them?

It's had a kind of paradoxical effect on me because although that was one of the most difficult things I've ever done and that was one of the hardest days of my life, it left me feeling very connected with people and very strong. And I didn't at all feel defeated because I felt like I had gone there, I had found them, I had come home, I had made it through the day without cutting. My therapist knew that I was going, and she said to me, "If you're going to go and if you find something, you need to call me." And so I talked to her. And there were other people I had been talking to before I went and when I got back. I was devastated, but it left me feeling like I can do this and it kind of gave me a renewed sense of motivation to do it. So, that lasted for a couple of weeks and then I shut down for a month. Then I cut myself.

I do feel like I've gotten a grip on things now. I feel like I had a slip and I have it under control, at least for now. But it does reinforce the idea that this is addicting for me and I need to be careful to take good care of myself because when I'm either unable or unwilling to do that, I revert back to cutting myself. And that's not what I want to do.

4 Self-Injuring Women at the Workplace

. . . .

Elizabeth: In the office . . . I always have to be careful of what I wear because I have to make sure that my scars or my cuts will be covered. I can't wear blouses that are going to show that I have a big bandage on my arm covering them up. People would see the gauze pads under the blouse and ask questions, so I always wear sweaters. But if it's hot and I'm wearing a sweater, I'm extremely hot. And sometimes I panic because I think, "Oh my gosh! What if I got so hot that I passed out and they took my sweater off?" This goes through my mind. I'm always thinking; I want to cover every single possibility.

One night I cut pretty bad . . . and my arm was sore and ended up getting infected. That affected me because I'm a typist at work and my arm hurt so badly. [That day] I stopped working and held my arm and someone walked by and said, "What's the matter?" I had to say, "Oh, nothing. I think I pulled a muscle or something." I wouldn't go to the doctor, and I know I needed stitches. I had to keep going into the bathroom and wiping off the blood, and changing the dressing because it bled constantly.

Then, of course, my mind wasn't where it should be — my mind was on *this*, and on the night before when I did it, and on that morning when I woke up with all the blood. I felt nauseous, and wasn't focusing at work, and people kept saying, "What's wrong with you? You seem really out of it today." People would say something to me and I'd be looking at them like I was listening, but I wouldn't hear a word they'd say, because I couldn't stay in the here and now. My day was totally off track — several days, actually.

One day I was sitting at my desk and this sweet, motherly woman came over. She was talking to me and she put her hand right on my arm and squeezed where I had cut the night before. I gasped, but I couldn't show her what was hurting. And I'm sitting there thinking, "Oh God, please let go of my arm," because I had an open gash, and it really hurt when she had her hand on it. But I couldn't say, "Can you remove your hand because it's hurting my arm." She would have said, "Why is it hurting your arm?" So I sat there and took it. My arm was throbbing. It's little things like that. People don't have a clue, but it's constantly there, always on my mind.

At work one time, I was cutting a bagel and I sliced the tip of my finger
with a knife — accidentally. I was kind of disappointed because it wasn't bad
enough. I didn't have any razor blades with me and the knife belonged to the
cafeteria, so I couldn't take it. So I took a paperclip and opened it, and I kept
going back and forth to the bathroom [to] stick the paperclip into the cut and
try to tear it open more. I was getting so aggravated because it . . . wasn't deep
enough, and I would try to pull my skin apart, trying to make it deeper. . . .

I get my work done, but on days that I cut, I'll go into work and won't talk
to a soul. They'll come up to me and say something like, "Are you depressed
today? You seem really depressed." And I'll say, "No, no, I'm fine, I'm fine." I
choose to cut myself off because I cut the night before and I'm totally numb.
I released everything that was built up inside and I feel emotionally numb
after it. . . . [But] it's not only a numbness from emotions, it's numbness from
everything. . . . I feel so numb I could sit in a chair and stare at the wall for
hours and hours and hours without blinking an eyelash. Those are the days I
can't talk to the people I work with because it's just not there. I'll totally focus
on my work, and sometimes if they say something to me, I don't even have
the energy to answer them. In that way, it affects my work big time because
then they see that and they're like, "What's wrong with *her*? Why is she so
quiet?" . . .

But I can get my work done. Once or twice I may not have done what I
needed to get done, but there's nobody breathing down my neck at work. It's
really an easygoing job which is great because I know I'm a good worker, but
we don't count our productivity; the work just gets done. I work well under
pressure. I shut myself off and I get into it, and I don't stop until I get it done.
I put deadlines on myself.

If [the cutting] were to affect my work at all it would not so much be in
doing less work, but doing more work because I put pressure on myself. I
don't want to have anything to do with what's going on around me and I need
something to focus on in order to be able to achieve that. I can do that with
my work. I can completely zone in on my work and I won't even hear a conversation that's going on at the next desk. I'll overachieve; I'll get double my
work done. If I feel like this and I'm cutting, I'll cut deep. And it's almost like
I'll work as hard as I would cut deep. If it's building up inside, I know that
focusing on my work will hold me over until I get home. Because when I get
home, I'll be able to cut. Knowing that, and knowing that the decision has
been made — "It's okay, once you're home, you can cut" — then I'm okay and
I can kind of ease up a little bit because I know that that's there for me. The
work will tide me over until I can leave, and go home and do what I really
want to do — which is cut. . . . Work is not a substitute, it's a temporary fill-in

until I can get where I can cut. It needs to be a private place, where no one knows this. . . .

I remember one time it was a high-stress morning. I was letting everything get to me. I didn't want to talk to the girls that I sit with. I just wanted to bury my head in my work and not talk to anybody. I remember that it was pretty early in the morning; I decided I'm going to cut. . . . Once I make that decision, it's there and I can't go back on it. It's almost like I give in to the decision that I've made, and I'm not going to fight it, because I don't have the energy to fight it. I'll get through my day thinking about it the whole time. It almost gives me a good feeling; it almost *helps* me because I say, "It's alright, I'll get rid of all this when I get home and I [can] cut." I'll drive home from work, planning out the whole thing. I'll go up to my room, change, and sit down and do it. And everything that I felt during the day will leave.

· · · · · · · · · ·

ELIZABETH DESCRIBES workdays permeated with the prelude or aftermath to self-cutting. Her day begins by putting on a cotton sweater no matter what the temperature outside, to adequately conceal scars, cuts, or bandages. She also must shield internal numbness, depression, obsessive thinking about past or planned self-cutting, and the physical pain her injured arm causes her. She partially succeeds, with her psychological turbulence revealed to colleagues only as quietness or depression, and her physical pain accepted as a "pulled muscle." "People don't have a clue, but it's constantly there, always on my mind." Throughout, she continues working, sometimes in frenzied concentration so as to neither think nor feel until she can get home and once again find release through cutting.

Like Elizabeth, other women who cut, burn, hit, or pick at themselves suffer from sometimes overpowering emotions, yet hold down responsible, part- or full-time jobs. In spite of occasional hospitalizations, periodic depressions, acute attacks of anxiety, multiple identities, or other signs of emotional distress, they keep on working.

The secrecy and misunderstanding surrounding self-injury make it seem incompatible with the requirements of the workplace. Consequently, "if they only knew" can be a recurring thought for self-injuring women at work: If they only knew that last night I cut myself, bled a lot, and am sitting with them now at this important meeting with my long sleeve pinned over the bandage so it won't show. If they only knew that I have several identities and the cutting is worse even though I'm totally on top of things here at work. If they only knew that I, the boss, cut myself, just as some of their clients do. If they only knew. . . .

Because of her working life, a woman who self-injures can feel split in two:

she is both the competent worker and the woman who does "bizarre" things and cannot stop.¹ She may feel fraudulent because of her hidden life behind the successful exterior.² As a worker she can be focused, organized, rational, intelligent, and sensible. She can be a sought-after professional who attains authoritative positions that entail planning, running meetings, directing agencies or businesses, and hiring, firing, and supervising staff. She can listen to coworkers' problems and let no one know of her own state of mind. She can become so absorbed in her work that she almost forgets that self-injury is a part of her life until, with dismay, she is reminded by a thought or action.

To make matters worse, self-injuring women know how others view self-injury. "I know [that cutting myself] sounds crazy, but I'm not a crazy person: I'm totally rational," Elizabeth said, protesting in advance any negative ideas I might have. "Part of me is sane," Edith said, speaking for other women who want it understood that self-injury does not negate their ability to function. They can be "two people" for years on end, with no one at work the wiser. They incorporate self-injury into their working lives so smoothly that no peers or subordinates suspect what they do to their bodies in order to function so well.

On the job, secrecy about self-injury can be paramount.³ "They don't know" or "They have no idea" are frequent replies about colleagues' or employers' reactions to self-injury. Clothing can usually cover most wounds and scars, and women who must come to work with visible self-inflicted sores or cuts can rely on colleagues' politeness in not asking questions. It is not polite to remark about the sore on a person's face or to question her explanation for needing bandages or crutches for her leg or foot. "They don't say anything, and I don't say anything," and business goes on as usual. For some women, the very idea of telling a colleague or employer about self-injury is appalling:

. . . .

Erica: I can't imagine anybody at work ever knowing this, I just can't imagine it. And I'm very friendly with people I work with now or have worked with. The company I used to work for has gone out of business, yet there's a whole group of us that gets together once a month for dinner — a nice circle of friends. And the woman I worked for on my previous job I now work for again; she recruited me away and we're friends. But I can't imagine ever telling any of them. I can't see that they would have any way to plug into it. . . .

For some of them I'm sure I'm the only lesbian they know. So it's always funny, you know, what am I going to tell them? Do I have to look like the perfect lesbian? You know, I have to be their shining example. . . . So I hesitate to tell them *anything* bad. I just don't see that they would know what to do with this. I think some of them have put together other parts of me that I've never explicitly told them, just like I've put together parts of them that they've never explicitly told me. I think if some of those things were to come up in conversation, that would work comfortably. But I can't imagine them talking about this. . . . There's no way to know who would react favorably, and the consequences are just too much to risk it. I mean, for all I know, a couple of them go home and do the same stuff! But there's no way to find out. . . .

. . . .

Among women who had not told an employer or colleague about self-injury, typical responses to the idea of disclosure were, "Oh, my God, I'd never tell my employer, never, never, never!" and "Ugh! I can't even imagine; I *cannot* imagine." Most women reacted with varying degrees of horror at the thought.[4] It would, they said, forever change the way their employers and colleagues saw them. "They would never be able to see me again in the same way" encapsulates most women's fears. Noting some colleagues' narrow views of anyone different from themselves, the women I interviewed consider a revelation of self-injury tantamount to an irreparable fall from grace:

. . . .

Erica: I have a reputation at work for being very capable, a quick learner, for being innovative in the way I approach problems — and I think all that would change. It's almost like alcoholics probably once were viewed many years ago: it was just not being able. . . . [Disclosing that I self-injure] would tend to color everything that they thought of me. I think *that* would become the defining characteristic of me for them. It immediately puts me in a different group and it would make them uncomfortable around me. It's not like saying to somebody, "I'm going to have my teeth bonded." "Oh, okay." It's a piece of information they file away and never think of again. Or, "You don't know this about me, but I only have nine toes," you know, something like that. "Well, that's an interesting new aspect. And how does that affect your life? Is it hard to buy shoes?" I just can't *see* me saying, "Well, you know, I cut myself with razor blades," and having them say, "Oh, how interesting! Tell me more. Gee, does that make it hard to buy short-sleeved blouses?" It's a dead-end conversation, and it's a bit of information that they're left with that they don't know what to do with. They've got nowhere to go to find out anything more about it: "What does this mean? Does this mean she's going to totally lose control some day and run through the office *slashing* people with razor blades? What does this mean? Does this mean that we can't trust her?" There's nothing to tell them what to do with this information.

. . . .

Even coworkers' knowledge of a woman's diagnosis, such as posttraumatic stress disorder, would not soften the impact of revealing self-injury, the lowest on the ladder of socially unacceptable conditions. "Weird," "impaired," "strange," and "sick" are some of the attributes that women fear would be permanently attached to their names. They fear that even their reputations as good workers would be forever tainted by disclosure of self-injury. Those who have difficult relations with employers would only be providing ammunition for more problems; and those for whom a small, tightly-knit office is like a family believe that this "family" would not understand self-injury.

In spite of all secrecy, however, some colleagues eventually find out. Often, a woman's hospitalization rather than her trust is the reason for disclosure. When a hospitalization forces a woman or a member of her family to reveal the whole or partial truth about her emotional health to someone at her workplace, self-injury can rapidly become common knowledge.

Disclosure is not always a painful experience. A gentle, caring, informed coworker who notices distress and will listen in times of turmoil is soothing on the job. It can be a relief not to have to be prepared with explanations and excuses if a wound or scar should show. An understanding colleague can discreetly relieve a woman from tasks such as opening packages that involve using a knife, thus helping her avoid temptations to cut herself at work. An informed colleague can prevent self-injury if an alter-identity has completely taken over a woman's actions at work and is about to cut in the colleague's presence. Some women have found valuable allies by choosing to disclose or through the forced disclosure of a hospitalization. A colleague or supervisor is sometimes an empathic person who will try to understand self-injury even if s/he does not condone it. Esther had just begun a job when she had to be hospitalized for a suicide attempt. When she came back to work, she said to her supervisor, "I understand totally if you don't want me to work here anymore. If I were in your shoes, I might not want me working here either." To her surprise, her supervisor said that she wanted her to continue working, giving Esther a much-needed sense of being accepted, of being okay. Similarly, Karen was praised for not bringing her emotional problems, whatever they might be, into the workplace. Her supervisor said that she valued Karen even though the supervisor realized that "there are things about you I don't know."

Fortunate is the woman whose coworker, supervisor, or employer has had personal experience with abuse and with the emotional problems that can follow. In such cases, mutual disclosure can be a pleasant experience, and even requesting a medical leave for a necessary hospitalization may elicit a benign "Do whatever you have to do. We'll deal with it." Women who have these experiences are aware of their rare good fortune in being able to safely reveal the truth about their scars or discuss their need for time off because of self-injury.

Nonetheless, there can be a price to pay for any allies won through disclosure. Some colleagues may be quietly afraid of self-injury, especially when it is coupled with multiple identities. Others, though well-meaning, may respond awkwardly:

. . . .

Esther: This one guy brought in something to be engraved, and it happened to be a very large knife that he used for scuba-diving and he asked if we could engrave it. I took it out of the sheath and I was looking at it to see what it was made of. And one of my coworkers came over and said, "I'll take care of this; you know how you are with knives." I said, "I can handle this," but she went ahead and [took it anyway].

. . . .

Here, Esther is treated like a child because her coworker, rather than respectfully asking Esther whether she would prefer having someone else engrave the knife, takes it from her, disregarding Esther's protest. Passing comments such as "That cut looks fresh, Esther!" may or may not feel accepting and acceptable. Colleagues may bring up the subject of self-injury when it is not necessary, or in an indiscreet, joking, or degrading manner when they do not know how to respond. When Esther has such experiences, they make her feel that other people neither respect what she is going through now nor understand what she has gone through in the past. Unfortunately, her feelings are probably based on fact: few colleagues are likely to understand the pain that underlies self-injury, an ignorance that itself can cause more pain for women who injure themselves. Esther perceives, however, that her colleagues' jokes reveal their nervousness about self-injury. Their sense of humor occasionally serves to relieve everyone's tension for a while, including her own.

Some women who have been hospitalized are not sure how disclosure has actually occurred. Theoretically, only a supervisor needs to know that a hospitalization is for emotional reasons. A supervisor sometimes chooses to protect a hospitalized woman by telling staff that the hospitalization is for a physical ailment (socially acceptable), rather than a psychological ailment (socially unacceptable). However, in a small group of coworkers, it is harder to be anonymous and secretive, and even harder if the small group lives in a small town:

. . . .

Karen: When something happens and I end up in the hospital, they won't question me about it. They might give me a hug or something, or they'll say,

"Are you alright?" and I'll say, "Yes." They never ask me what happened and I usually don't volunteer it. There's only one [colleague] that I have actually talked with about it at any length and that's because her daughter cuts and I think that she can understand. I think they're afraid of it; they don't understand it; it freaks them out. I can't really help them to understand, so I don't try. They just think I'm a little off the wall. I let them think that; I don't know how to make them think anything else.

. . . .

When secrecy is preserved at the workplace, it is usually due to the extreme taboo of self-injury, not to poor relationships with colleagues. Most of the women I talked with get along well with their colleagues, although relationships vary from the friendly but distant, to those who go out socially with colleagues. Nonetheless, self-injury subtly or overtly affects most women's collegial relationships. Jane, an already shy woman, avoids her coworkers more than usual when she has just cut, fearing to reveal her emotions. Karen, who has friendly, caring relationships with coworkers, nonetheless senses a certain reservation among colleagues who know about the self-injury or about unspecified emotional problems. For Elizabeth, friendly relationships become troublesome when coworkers show their care partly by observing her and commenting on her perennial long-sleeves or a scar that happens to show beneath a sleeve pushed up absentmindedly in the heat of summer.

Collegiality can suffer even more during the warm months of the year when company outings tempt a scarred woman to the pool- or lakeside. Pleased by the prospect, a woman may originally accept, only to have to refuse the invitation when she remembers what a bathing suit or even short sleeves will reveal. Forced to isolate herself from her colleagues, she may make them wonder at her repeated refusals. Only if a woman is certain that there will be no word said, no furtive glances, no questions, no whisperings, no awareness whatsoever of her scars, could she feel comfortable at such an event. As she knows, these are impossible expectations.

Self-Injury on the Job

In spite of self-injury's presence as a secret or revealed factor in these working women's lives, it has little effect on their productivity. Only Jane and Elizabeth said that their ability to work is affected by self-injury or by scars. For Jane, the only effect is an adjustment in an already flexible schedule. When she has just cut and her emotions are still high, she does not go to work unless she knows that she can work by herself so that no one will observe her emotional state.

In contrast, Elizabeth's workdays are sometimes dominated by the pain and blood of a deep wound that has to be hidden and surreptitiously tended. Her work time is also affected by frequent trips to the bathroom to change the dressing of a prior cut, to secretly self-injure, or to go to the hospital for stitches. However, the problem that has the greatest impact on Elizabeth at work is the uncontrollable and overwhelming nature of the feelings that can lead to cutting. Yet, in spite of everything, Elizabeth usually gets her work done. The need to cut even improves her productivity because the same negative feelings that eventually lead to cutting make her avoid all contact with her coworkers. Complete absorption in her work is a way of avoiding contact, and she will "work as hard as I would cut deep."

In fact, my informants suffer from their work far more than their work suffers from self-injury.[5] The stress of any job, new or old, can cause some women to injure themselves more frequently. The additional learning often necessary for a new job can make a woman feel incompetent, lost, and dependent, especially if she sets stricter standards for herself than for others. Such feelings can lead to self-injury as a form of self-chastisement as well as a necessary release from emotions. Some jobs seem created to induce stress so severe that it encourages some form of explosion:

. . . .

Erica: When I was working for newspapers I had a job that was very frustrating because I had to deal with editors and production people at different levels and try to get them to work together to produce this newspaper. They had very different goals in mind and I was in the middle. That was my job: keeping them separate and making them work together. I had a different deadline every ten minutes all morning long. And I would go into the locker room with big thick walls, and just bash my head against the wall, trying to adjust, trying to step out of it. It was really like going into the back room and having a shot of whiskey: it kind of calms you down, steadies the nerves — at least temporarily.

. . . .

Being solely in charge of a large group or organization can feel like a reenactment of a traumatic childhood situation: being pushed to and beyond one's limits with no help or resources. Feeling alone with one's work and unsupported by coworkers can also remind a woman of situations when she hid from her family and was alone. If there is no time to look for other work, a woman can feel trapped in her situation, just as she did as an abused child. Her work then becomes a "flashback of the past," as Barbara calls it. Even if a woman realizes that her current situation is not the same as her past abuse, the resemblance can add even more stress to the load she already bears. Eventually, the self-injury caused by work-related stress may force a woman to leave her job before she has found another position.

At the job, release from the stress of work often cannot tolerate any delay. Chastisement from a supervisor can lead to high anxiety and the need for instant calming. Worry about a project can require quick release. Habitual overwork with unusually long hours and no break can lead to the need for soothing and relief. A little bit of cutting in the bathroom; the quick picking at a scab to feel the blood; a hand under the conference table digging a thumb-tack into the skin: these acts can enable a woman to get through the stress of the moment and stay on the job.

Brief episodes of self-injury at work enable a woman to keep working and get through the day as a functioning person. Women describing their self-injury at the workplace have a recurring theme: ". . . and then I go back to work." I flick off a scab, and then I go back to work; I go into the bathroom and cut, and then I go back to work; I bang my head against the wall, and then I go back to work. Such episodes take place under the noses of coworkers, supervisors, or employers who are oblivious to a woman's self-injuring acts but sometimes uncomfortably close to discovery:

· · · · · · · · ·

Edith: I remember one time — and it was so embarrassing and so weird —
[at work] I pulled off the skin [around one of my fingernails], and it started bleeding. *Just* after I did that somebody came around the corner and wanted to talk to me   we were both standing. I realized that it was bleeding inside my hand so I held my hand down and it started bleeding onto the floor while I was talking to this guy. And somehow, when we were done he noticed the blood on the floor and said, "Where did *that* come from?" And I said, "Gee, I don't know," and I was sort of holding my hand. It was one of those things where if I'd been caught at it I would have been embarrassed, ashamed, mortified.

　　　　　　　　　　　　　　　　　· · · · · · · · · ·

Women I spoke with who self-injure in response to situations at work describe their jobs as highly stressful.[6] Trapped at work, yet with a strong need for release, a woman feels that she has no option but to injure herself at work or to use her lunch break to briefly flee:

· · · · · · · · ·

Barbara: Sometimes people would have lunch together and I knew that I'd need to be alone. So I'd run to my car. There were days that I'd drive down the block and cut, but there were other days that I'd shut the windows and scream or cry or just breathe. Then I didn't have to cut because I'd at least tuned in and was there for me.

. . . .

Caught in a lengthy meeting, a woman may find ways to surreptitiously calm herself, such as sliding an earring up her sleeve and digging it into her arm, telling herself, "Okay, I'm going to get through this." Sitting in a cubicle at her desk with her back to the door, she can quickly pick at a sore, scratch her skin, or even cut the cuticles off her nails to find relief without blood. Always she is careful not to make any movement that would give away her secret soothing. A woman may even come to work with a safety pin already fastened to her skin beneath her shirt sleeves, prepared for whatever may come. Rubbing her arm a bit at work heightens the pin's effects and is an innocuous gesture that can be done in full view of her colleagues.

Nonetheless, among my informants, self-injury was never disabling unless it escalated to a point at which a woman needed to stop work and get help. Barbara is the only one of my informants who eventually felt compelled to leave her job because stress was causing intolerable self-injury: ". . . thirteen stitches here and ten stitches there; it was getting pretty bad that I had to do that to get through the day."

Yet, women self-injure on the job not only because of work stress, but also because it is too difficult to get through a whole day without it. Even when work is not highly stressful, the thoughts, memories, and emotions that a woman must live with can cause her to self-injure during working hours. Several women spoke of the ways in which their secret actions help them through their working days. For example, pervasive anxiety can require repeatedly seeing or feeling blood:

. . . .

Edith: There have been times when I've been treating a patient and maybe I have something [to pick] on my leg. And I'll pick at it and then realize that it's going to bleed through my pants. . . . If I'm wearing black pants I don't worry about it—it's so complicated, and so screwy. Let's say the person is lying on the bed and I've just shown them an exercise that I want them to do. I can be sitting in a chair and pick in a way that they can't see. There's a spot on my leg right now. If I leaned down like this and picked, you would never know, and I could have picked the scab off. Sometimes I've wanted to pick while I've been seeing a patient and I haven't and then I'll get out to the car and it's like, "I *have* to do this."

• • •

Rosa: I have exacto knives and sometimes I'll give myself a little nick. I have this zit on my face and I've been picking that at work. I'll move my hand across my face and do it real fast. I turn my back towards the door and pretend like I'm really concentrating on something.

· · · · · · · · · ·

Other powerful feelings or the internal voices of alter identities saying unbearable things can have the same effect:

· · · · · · · · ·

Esther: For a while, I had a razor blade hidden in the ladies room and I would use that. Also, I have a razor knife in my desk drawer. . . . I go to the ladies room, I don't know what it is, I don't feel it; I just kind of go into a trance almost and I take the razor blade or knife and put it against my skin and push down and drag it across my skin until blood comes out. . . . I let it bleed and look at it for a while, and then I clean it up. If it needs a bandage, I put a band-aid on it. Then I go back to work.

· · · · · · · · · ·

Work requiring a woman to be alone with little to do can trigger self-injury simply because it offers few distractions from thoughts and memories, not usually pleasant company for an abused woman. With time on her hands, her thoughts can build up and become painful obsessions difficult to bear. Esther, whose evening work situation in a store is often quiet and lonely, sometimes finds herself with a shipment of knives that she is required to engrave, an almost diabolical invitation to cut away all negative thoughts and emotions.

Even with plenty to occupy one's mind and with coworkers around, resistance to invitations such as easily accessible knives and razor blades can be difficult. Many jobs involve work with sharp instruments, tempting self-injury that would look like an accident. Such an "accident" would, however, attract attention to the injury, usually the last thing a self-injuring woman wants.

Fearful of attracting attention or of going too far, a woman may try not to injure herself until she leaves work. Instead, she will soothe herself by taking time out to call an informed and trusted person such as a therapist or local rape crisis center, or by thinking about how she will injure herself once she gets home: "It's okay; once you're home, you can cut." If she has resisted throughout the day, as soon as she pulls out of her office parking lot she may turn onto a side street, park, and injure herself, so urgent is her need for release.

Career Boundaries

Self-injury can contribute to feelings of unworthiness, acting as a constant reminder to an abused woman that she is "not good enough" and preventing her from achieving her full career potential. Self-injury may also sap a woman's energy and thus keep her from expanding all her horizons, including her career horizons. She may not have her mind free enough to think about the future, or may not feel that she has a future. Being in a "survival mode" does not encourage a woman to further her career. Even a woman who is trying to stop self-injury may find that the daily struggle to restrain herself is draining energy she could be putting into her life, including her work. Barbara said that when she first stopped taking drugs, she felt free to function at a more productive level. She wants to reach that point of liberation from cutting as well in order to feel autonomous, empowered, and motivated to rise above hindrances.

Scars and self-injury have not prevented my informants from taking advantage of job offers, but self-injury can affect career directions or job choices. Any job that requires wearing a bathing suit, such as work involving swimming with a client as part of therapy, can be out of bounds for a woman with scars on her arms or legs. Work requiring a short-sleeved uniform is either unacceptable or demands a willingness to be questioned, a plausible lie, and no fresh wounds on the arms. A woman with scratches or cuts on her hands can feel that the medical profession is not an option for her, even though gloves are a routine requirement. Working among therapists can be hard to accept if it entails discussing the consequences of childhood abuse and thus feels "too close to home."

Some women who self-injure may be subtly guided in their choice of professions by their past experiences. One survey suggests that the most frequent choices of profession among women who self-injure are teacher and nurse.[7] However, caregiving (both paid and unpaid) is a traditional role for women and thus may explain any such career-choice trends for women who self-injure. It is striking that among my fifteen informants, five are current or aspiring social or human service workers. One possible explanation is the wish to help other victims, a wish perhaps guided by the knowledge that unique understanding and empathy can come from having similarly suffered.

Self-injuring women who work in the mental health field might expect to find greater understanding of self-injury among their colleagues. Like people from other professions, however, mental health professionals can be relatively ignorant and judgmental about self-injury, and the ignorant and knowledgeable alike may feel unease, disdain, or revulsion. Even those with more understanding can be horrified at the idea that a woman who self-injures might cross the boundary from client ("patient") to colleague. Jessica, who is working as an intern in psychiatric social work while going back to school, finds such boundaries difficult — perhaps impossible — to cross:

. . . .

I think the self-injury is very unacceptable. I have a lot of difficulty already because they want to make clear distinctions in who should be a therapist and who should be a client. That's part of what the labels are doing, especially with "borderline": it's okay if you're a client, but it's not okay if you're a therapist — it's not okay if you're a *peer*. When they're treating borderlines they want them to be treated decently in the world. When they actually meet one, they don't want her to be a peer. So, given that there's so much flack that I've gotten already just with saying that I'm a survivor . . . saying that I have been diagnosed borderline and multiple is just throwing me out. If anybody there finds out that I self-injure, it's over, and always will be. If I do manage to become a therapist, I'll probably always have the potential of destroying my career if it becomes known that I self-injure.

. . . .

A mental health worker who self-injures can find herself in painful situations. She may overhear colleagues discussing a client who self-injures. As Peggy says, "I hear things sometimes. I realize they could be talking about me." She may feel self-conscious, as though the therapists might somehow divine that she injures herself. Meredith and Peggy have had to listen to colleagues' insulting remarks about clients, such as "She's just doing that for attention" or "Oh, that's so gross!" Meredith notices the amazement in their voices — "How can she not *feel* that?" — referring to the painless self-cutting she herself knows so well. Barbara once found herself in the ironic position of going with her colleagues to a workshop on self-injury. While her colleagues dutifully took notes, she sat next to them thinking, "I've been there; I've done that; I understand it from the inside out."

A self-injuring woman may also feel an advantage over her colleagues in knowledge, understanding, and empathy — an advantage she cannot easily discuss or try to share. When asked at a job interview about her knowledge of drug and alcohol addiction, Barbara, crossing the boundary between therapist and client, courageously referred to her own past problems as part of her credentials: "I've also done a lot of field work in this. I've been in recovery from drug and alcohol use for quite a while." She thinks that all her experiences, including self-injury, are valuable for her as a social worker.

Barbara, who is secure in her job, also once disclosed her self-injury at work to educate her subordinates. She was supervising a group of mental health workers who had a "them versus us" mentality toward their clients, which aggravated Barbara. When she finally told them about her self-injury, a shocked and awkward silence followed, leading her to feel somewhat ambivalent about having disclosed this secret in a state of frustration and anger:

. . . .

People act like they're so much different than the clients. I don't think it's a good attitude that clinicians take, and so I sometimes have outed myself about different things. If they accept me already at the workplace and they're thinking that these things [only] happen to other people, I'll just say, "Well, I did that." Whether they're making fun of the client or they're just outraged that the clients are sexually promiscuous, I'll say, "I used to be like that." Or if they say, "Oh no, this person's smoking pot; he'll do any drug that's around," I say, "I used to be like that." And when we're talking about cutting, they just say, "I don't get it. Who in their right mind would be slicing their own body up? You have to be pretty sick to do that. . . ." And I was like, "Hey, plenty of people who are out there functioning in the world are cutters. Many people do it and you don't even know. Like me, for instance; I had a regular habit of cutting myself, and I couldn't stop." I just wanted to educate them about it—that it doesn't mean you're a total loser.

. . . .

Barbara stands among other mental health professionals who have disclosed their past self-injury.[8] Some of them feel obliged to be honest in order to prepare the way for other currently or formerly self-injuring professionals.

Being a mental health colleague as well as a mental health client makes a woman feel that there is little difference between the two, a feeling that contrasts sharply with some of her colleagues' perceptions of clear distinctions and impenetrable boundaries between colleague and client. Yet, different kinds of problems may arise when a woman who self-injures works with clients who injure themselves. If the shorter, thinner sleeves of a hot summer reveal a counselor's scars to a client, will the revelation change the client/counselor relationship? If so, for better or for worse? Will the client simply think, "Oh good, someone really understands." Or will the client want to discuss the counselor's problem or worry about provoking her into further self-injury? Barbara, who faced this situation, decided that although her personal experiences are an asset, they should not detract from her job as a professional whose responsibility is to discuss her clients' problems: "If they asked [about my scars], I'd probably say, "We're here to talk about *you*. You don't need to worry about me."

Working toward Change

American workplaces have become more tolerant of differences that once were taboo. Though men may tell sexist jokes among themselves, many men now know better than to tell them with impunity at work. Snide remarks about homosexuality, race, or religion are no longer publicly tolerated, nor is job discrimination on the basis of these factors. Some companies have strong policies of tolerance and diversity, and some now offer medical benefits to "domestic partners," a policy unthinkable in the recent past. Mental health problems and coping strategies such as self-injury, however, remain deprived of broad public understanding and acceptance.

Can the workplace become a place more tolerant of self-injury? Theoretically, at a workplace where employers and colleagues accept a variety of races, religions, and sexual preferences, one could be honest about self-injury. In many workplaces, however, tolerance for diversity does not yet include tolerance for emotional problems. As Mary said, "I see a lot of groups of people that meet at work, but I sure don't see any for emotional problems."

Women who injure themselves want the kind of tolerance that can come through positive exposure to people who look or behave differently. Yet, understandably, none of my informants could conceive of comfortably revealing their self-injury in their own workplaces solely to further this goal:

. . . .

Erica: I guess some things can start in the workplace, I'm just not sure how. I'm so invested in this being not known that I can't imagine it being known. There's enough public perception about almost anything else you can name, even right down to being an extraterrestrial, that you can picture workplaces saying, "Oh, wow, that's interesting" or "I know where you can get help for that." Either they're going to be intrigued by it, or eager to help you work it out. But this—I think people would just be knocked into silence. I don't see how it could happen in the workplace. There must be something else that I could think back to that was this important to keep hidden. You would think that somebody who lost a job because she was lesbian would have an immediate answer for that, but it doesn't feel the same. I wasn't as invested in keeping that hidden—I *wasn't* keeping it hidden. I just chose to tell the truth selectively, which is, I guess, what I continue to do with [self-injury]: I talk to you; I talk to my therapist; I talk to my partner and a few, selected friends. It's very selective truth-telling: my boss has no idea; my coworkers have no idea; people I see all the time have no idea. If this room [where just the two of us are talking privately] was *full* of women who did the same stuff, and we sat here for a couple of hours and had a really wonderful talk, could I walk out there and tell [my colleagues] what we had been talking about? No.

.   .   .   .

In many cases, disclosure at the workplace would be damaging to women's careers because of too little public knowledge and support. Until large-scale public discussion of the issue exists, women who self-injure are caught in workplace environments that cannot be safely changed, and self-injury will not be acknowledged at the workplace as an unfortunate but temporarily useful way of coping.

Some women like to think that compassionate work policies can eventually be stretched far enough to include self-injury. Esther, whose problems are already known at her workplace, is beginning the process of change with informal "consciousness-raising" on her own:

.   .   .   .

We have this new rule in our office that if you are out of work for a doctor's appointment for half a day, then you can count that as a sick day. If I take a half of [a] day to go to therapy, I can't take that as a sick day; I have to take that as half of a vacation day. I don't think that it's fair. . . . There was another coworker who had cancer, and I feel badly that she had cancer. She had to take many days off for follow-up check-ups, which she had taken as sick days. I had an appointment at two in the afternoon and I said to my supervisor, "I'm going to take two hours of sick time." And she said, "What?" and I said, "I have a therapy appointment." And she said, "That'll have to be vacation time." "No, no, no, it's health." She goes, "Yes, but that's *mental* health." "Oh well, is it going to be different if I cut my wrist? Are you going to allow me to take it as sick time then?" And she said, "Are you trying to threaten me?" "No, I'm just trying to make you aware of what you're saying."

.   .   .   .

Esther and other women have constructive ideas about changes needed in the workplace, including ways that the workplace could be less likely to encourage self-injury. Some suggestions for achieving this goal are the same changes that women, especially mothers, have been fighting for years to obtain. These attributes would help transform any workplace into an environment that shows at least as much care and respect for the worker as for the work. The requirement of "reasonable accommodation" in the *Americans with Disabilities Act*[9] could be cited to implement some of these suggestions:

1. *Flextime* gives a woman a sense of autonomy and control, so necessary to the emotional health of us all. For a woman who injures herself, flextime

would allow her to set her own schedule for therapy appointments or for other needs for herself or her children. Of course, flexibility should not be attached to insufficient wages or benefits.

2. *Working as a team* in which members take care of and respect each other can keep a woman from feeling isolated, overwhelmed, or without options or control.

3. The opportunity for occasional, brief periods of *privacy* can make the difference between resorting to or averting self-injury.

4. An *available and helpful supervisor* can lower work-related stress, thereby lowering a woman's need to self-injure.

5. *Time out* for lunch and for brief morning and afternoon intervals of relaxation can help subdue any mounting tension.

6. *Sick time* rather than vacation time for therapy appointments and for any upsetting aftermath of therapy is a much-needed acknowledgment that mental health problems are as important and worthy of treatment as physical illnesses.

7. A *leave policy* that guarantees a return to work after a period of incapacitation can relieve the added stress of worrying about one's job and finances while trying to regain emotional stability.

8. In large corporations, where support groups are often offered only for alcohol and other drug abuses, *support groups* could provide confidential help for all emotional problems.

9. An *understanding and compassionate employee-assistance person* with whom a woman can consult openly and honestly can help allay work-related crises before they become too difficult to settle in healthful ways.

Currently, self-injuring women work with little or no workplace support and no acknowledgment of the courage required to lead a structured, productive life in the face of sometimes massive emotional pain. Many formerly abused women are able to be productive members of the workforce partly because self-injury allows them to cope with the emotional aftermath of abuse. Yet, their coping strategy is itself a taboo at the workplace, an environment that can mimic women's past abuse and increase their need to self-injure. Implementing the changes listed above would be a gesture of admiration for self-injuring women's courage and productivity, as well as an offer of concrete help.

5 *Life with Lovers, Families, and Friends*

AMONG WOMEN abused during childhood, self-injury begins as the outcome of a problem in a relationship: an older person, usually an adult, behaves toward the child in physically, sexually, or psychologically harmful ways that violate the child's trust and often her body. When the abuser is a caregiver or other family member, a child's love, dependence, and desire to please are neglected or misused. Among my informants, all but Helena were abused as children by a parent or stepparent, and two of Helena's three abusers were family members. Not surprisingly, abuse and self-injury leave emotional trails that affect these women's relationships as adults.

If sexual abuse was part of a woman's past experiences, physical intimacy in adulthood can be problematic, even impossible:

. . . .

Edith: One of the awful things that my father did was that he would turn me on as a little kid, so that I would *want* to do it. Now, I can't even put "normal" and "sexual relationship" in the same sentence. I don't want sex with anybody, man or woman. Whether or not I will ever have a "normal" sexual life is up for grabs. I suppose that would be the final accomplishment: to be able to have pleasurable sex with somebody.

. . . .

As Edith's experience suggests, prior abuse, current emotions, and secrecy combine to make it unusually difficult for a woman who self-injures to establish relationships of physical affection and trust. This can be true even for women with long-term partners. Because of past abuse, a woman's emotional responses can be numbed in continuous self-defense. She may loathe her body, be unwilling to have her feelings or her body exposed to another person, and find the idea of sex revolting. When looking at women friends who have sex, some traumatized women cannot imagine what such a life would be like. The only associations they have with sex are fear and shame.

A woman who self-injures may also have other signs of sexual revulsion, such as believing that her sexual anatomy is abnormal or feeling that she would be better off without a vagina. Although some women who are greatly afraid of sex do have occasional sexual relationships, they may do so only under coercion. Even if they feel desirous and pursue a lover, their negative feelings after having sex often act as punishment for any pleasure they may have had:

. . . .

Edith: It took my boss months to get to the point where I had sex with him. But he would turn me on, you know, a little petting, and it would get a little bit further, and a little bit further. So, I'd get turned on by the sex and do it, and then be afraid afterwards—in remembering what I had done. In my mind it equated with any old capital offense that you could think of: murder, pillage, rape—it felt so bad that *I* had done it. And this is one of the things that I "know" is a normal human activity and that people do it and it's supposed to be pleasurable and enjoyable—but *not* for me. For me, it's terrifying.

. . . .

Because of their feelings about sex with men, some heterosexual women think that they may be lesbians, only to discover that they do not want to make love with women, either. Some lesbian women also find that they do not want to have sex. As a result, some women who self-injure choose long-term celibacy as the only acceptable option.

A woman who self-injures as a result of emotional rather than physical abuse may feel no sexual revulsion, yet fear close sexual involvements because of disclosure: her secret might have to be revealed. Reluctance to entrust anyone with this secret, or to trust anyone at all, can deter a woman from seeking a serious emotional involvement. Some women have disclosed to a sexual partner, only to have her or him withdraw as a result, adding to their fear of becoming involved again. Others have had such experiences in their imaginations:

. . . .

Peggy: I feel like if I started to really care about somebody and they saw this, they'd probably go running as fast as they possibly could in the opposite direction. It's hard for me to imagine that somebody would want to deal with this.

. . . .

A woman who has injured herself for years and is now trying to stop may be ambivalent about an intimate relationship at this stage in her recovery. Barbara's past partners, for example, have been men, then women, all of whom were alcoholics or who self-injured. Now, if she should become sexually involved again, she would want a relationship with a person in recovery or one who has never been afflicted with such problems. Yet, because of the great shame she feels when she does have a fresh scar, she does not feel ready for a relationship based on recovery: "You know, you can hide scars pretty good even in bathing-suit weather; you can cut where your bathing suit covers. But if you are in a love relationship, they see all of you." Living with someone might deprive her of the privacy to cut if she felt the need, or even cause her to cut to have an excuse to remain clothed and say "no" to the intimacy she actually fears.

Given their past histories, the number of my informants who have partners and children is remarkable. Nonetheless, all but one of the women who are now or once were heterosexual and who have been sexually abused experience sexual problems.[1] They speak of infrequent or unwilling sex and of "good, healthy, sexual feelings" as a rarity:

. . . .

Elizabeth: [My fiance] had known about my past sexual issues and he was trying to be understanding, but then on the other hand he wasn't. He had kept his distance from me. But when I came back [after having left him], he said, "Well, I know that you have problems with your past, but I have physical needs, and I need sex, so we're going to have sex." It was like a condition of our relationship. [I felt] used, dirty.

The night I came back to him he said, "Oh, I have a surprise for you, something really special." It was this awful, trashy lingerie. It made me feel cheap. He wasn't even buying it for me, he was buying it for himself. I felt like he was expecting me to perform for him. It made me feel like I felt when I was a little girl: out of control, scared because I couldn't stop what was happening. . . .

Sometimes I thought I would want to [have sex with my fiance], but when it would start, I would get scared. I felt like I was fifteen again, and it was my brother. I never felt anything, and [my fiance] never could see that. He always used to say, "Wasn't that *great*, honey?" I think it might have been different if he had been a little more considerate, but he was selfish sexually, where it was all for him.

When we were together and we were about to have sex, he always undressed me. Even though it was only me and him, I felt like I was being exposed. Sometimes I'd block my mind, and I wouldn't think about it; I would just go along with it. But I never felt like I was really there. It's like I just pulled away, and then I went on autopilot, and I would just go with what was happening.

. . . .

Here, Elizabeth describes having to relive her past with someone she had hoped would be part of her future. Sex is an ordeal she endures partly by dissociating: she uses the tried-and-true method of separating her mind from her body, a "lovemaking" technique she shares with other women—heterosexual and lesbian alike—who have experienced sexual abuse.

Self-injury and visible scars can add to sexual unease. A woman who cuts her breasts and vagina is saying something about her feelings concerning sex, something that may or may not convey itself to her partner. Also, wounds or scars can affect the way a woman feels about her body and about her own attractiveness, possibly increasing her unwillingness to expose her body to her partner, making any physical intimacy unwanted and, at times, virtually extinguishing her sexual desire. A new partner's initial reaction to wounds or scars can be a litmus test: the partner must notice the wounds, yet accept and desire the person.

Whether a scar is old or new can make a difference. For women in long-term relationships, old scars may no longer be problematic and may never have caused concern. Fresh cuts, more visible than the old, can remind a woman of how she felt while cutting, feelings not at all conducive to lovemaking. Also, the sight of a new scar can provoke a partner's fear or anger and destroy any relaxed desire for intimacy:

. . . .

Rosa: [In] my previous relationship, at first the sex was really good. Then she started picking on me about housework and about "Why do you do this to yourself?" and I felt no desire. I couldn't be intimate with her, and the more she picked on me about what I did, the more I would pick on myself. Then there would be more active scars and she would say that she didn't want to touch me, and I would feel more dirty and ashamed.

. . . .

The intimacy of sharing a bedroom and of making love can enable a woman's partner to discover fresh scars. Some women know that their partners surreptitiously look at them, watching for new signs of self-injury:

. . . .

Jane: My husband has watched me while I was asleep to see if he could notice any new marks without actually embarrassing me by asking me.

. . .

Erica: She doesn't *like* it. I can see her checking out every little mark sometimes. See, these [scratches] are legitimately from gardening, but the other day I could see her checking them out, trying to decide: "Should I ask about them?" . . . I could watch her face doing this; it was really annoying.

. . . .

If a woman does not want her partner to know that she has recently self-injured, her effort to hide new scars may further inhibit lovemaking. One solution is to put on a long-sleeved nightgown and keep it on while making love, as Jane does. However, clothing can also arouse suspicion:

. . . .

Erica: I think what's more a problem is not so much scars as bruises or little cuts. The kinds [of things] that don't really leave scars and that go away in a couple of weeks—those things that I don't want her to see. She said to me the other night, "Why are you sleeping in pajamas? You never used to sleep in pajamas." And I could tell that what she was getting at was, "What are you hiding from me?" That was awkward; that was hard. In that way I'm always double-checking. I think, "Is she going to notice anything?"

. . . .

Self-injury and its resulting scars can be a source of turmoil within sexual partnerships.[2] When the partnership is a marriage, husbands may tend to view self-injury as reflections upon themselves: either they feel blamable for not being able to stop their wives' self-injury, or they think that they cause it. According to Jane, her husband thinks that her cutting is his failure. "What more can I do?" he asks. "What more can I do to help you or protect you?" He confiscates razors that Jane buys and supervises any blades she may need for household projects, treating her, through his concern, like a child. Although he still tries to control Jane's access to sharp objects, he has recently realized that nothing he does can prevent Jane from injuring herself.

Esther says that her husband responds to her self-injury as though she had just cut him instead of herself. "Don't you know how much this hurts me?" he asks, a reaction that makes Esther feel ashamed and even more secretive about her cutting. He also thinks that he is somehow the cause of her self-injury. "Do I depress you that much that you have to cut yourself?" he asks, showing his misunderstanding of self-injury despite Esther's attempts to explain it.

Esther finds her husband's responses an additional burden, although she realizes that part of what he feels is fear that she might cut herself progressively deeper, eventually committing suicide. Esther, like Jane, has tried to kill herself, and both husbands associate self-cutting with suicide. Nonetheless, his way of expressing himself actually lacks genuine concern for Esther's welfare:

"Don't you understand what this is doing to me, knowing that you cut yourself or knowing that you want to die? You *can't* die; don't you know the kids need you?" Jane does not find her husband's behavior an added stress because she understands that his reactions stem from his love for her. Instead, she is concerned that self-injury has repeatedly eroded her husband's trust in her, a trust she wants to maintain.

Like Jane, Karen was also once concerned that her husband would think her untrustworthy if she cut. She now realizes that it is not possible to promise her husband never to cut again, and when she cuts she no longer feels that she has broken his trust. True trust, she says, has to come from sharing the experience of cutting and its aftermath.

Unmarried women in sexual relationships also find that self-injury brings some degree of turmoil with the partners in their lives. Erica has a partner of twelve years, a woman who is concerned, caring, and empathetic. Nonetheless, the two have negotiated and quarreled over Erica's possession of razor blades at their home. Erica's partner feels reassured by the fact that Erica considers self-injury "not good" and talks about it with a therapist. For her own part Erica is grateful, despite conflicts, to finally have an empathetic partner, after experiencing partners who distanced themselves upon disclosure, or who betrayed Erica's secret to a third person.

Rosa, too, is grateful. Between our interview sessions, Rosa's lover disclosed that she had injured herself a few times during a period of depression after simultaneously losing her lover, her house, her job, and her dog. Rosa's response was astonishment at finding out that this woman, so close to her, once injured herself. "I just said, 'Wow, this is so amazing,' because she has been real supportive and now I can understand a little bit more why she's been so supportive."

For Elizabeth, self-injury became a reason to cancel her plans for marriage. She could not make her fiance understand why she cuts herself, and she did not actually want to make him a confidant. "[The cutting] was helping me, and he couldn't see that, and no one else can see that." Partly because Elizabeth kept this important part of her life to herself, her partner felt insecure in the relationship. Possibly he also associated self-cutting with suicide, increasing his misunderstanding and suspiciousness. As Elizabeth tells it, she finally had to make a major choice concerning her future. She did not waver in her decision:

. . . .

For me, it's a coping mechanism; it helps me to deal with stuff. And the problems that we were having in our relationship, the cutting was a coping

mechanism for them, too. It becomes a coping mechanism for almost everything that comes up. . . . He didn't understand that—which a lot of people
don't. He thought I could just stop, just like that, and that I could trust him,
which I couldn't do. The cutting was becoming harder and harder to hide
from him because of the sexual relationship. So the more he would notice
and point it out and get angry, the more shame I would feel and the more
angry I would get at him for pointing it out and at me for doing it. And it
made me pull away from him. I almost felt like he was forcing me to trust
him. So, it was either trust in him, stop cutting just like that—which I
couldn't do anyway—and find other ways, or leave him. So I left him. That
wasn't the sole reason I left him, but it was a big part of it. [I had to choose
between him and cutting], and I did choose. Because, if you laid the two out
on the table—in my mind, he wasn't helping [me] cope with anything. The
cutting was, and is. So, which one would *you* choose?

. . . .

Elizabeth's logic is irrefutable: what helps one cope in life wins, unless an
equally successful substitute can be found.

Rosa's former lover was initially understanding about self-injury but the
understanding was not deep. Instead, it became the familiar refrain: "If you
don't want to do this anymore, just stop!" Thus, the partner's empathy became
controlling and abusive, reminding Rosa of her relationship with her father.
"I felt like a little kid. I felt like I wanted to please her and get her approval, so
I stopped." Rosa agreed to stop self-injuring at the end of a three-month "recovery" period, an arrangement she now realizes was absurd. After stopping
for a while, Rosa injured herself more severely than ever when her demanding
lover left her.

Of the women I interviewed who have ever had long-term male partners,
only Jane seems to see her partner as an ally, of sorts, concerning self-injury.
Although Jane tries to hide her self-injury from her husband, she conveys the
picture of a loving partnership and of her knowledge that his reactions to self-
injury stem from love and care. Almost all other heterosexual women give the
impression that their partners' responses are stressful and that the relationship itself is occasionally a source of major stress. For two women, the stress of
the relationship sometimes leads to self-injury. Among the six actively lesbian
women, four have been in relationships with women who were not empathetic, and three have harmed themselves due to the stress of the relationship.

Do the self-injuring women's relationships described here and on the preceding pages say anything about female versus male partners' responses to self-

injury? First, several women mentioned that their male partners felt obliged to "do something" in response to self-injury. These men may not know what to do and search for appropriate action when only empathy is called for. Consequently, they may feel inadequate and become frustrated and angry at their own inability to stop a partner's self-injury. Second, many women have been in situations in which they felt that a heterosexual experience was like rape. In contrast, female partners are probably better able to intuit the long-term effects of repeated sexual violations. Even when a man is raped as a boy, his experience is different from a girl's experience, although such a man may have more empathy for rape victims of both sexes. Third, men's friendships often have a different basis than women's and do not necessarily include discussion of personal problems, fears, or perceived "weaknesses," discussions that would provide opportunities to practice empathy. All these factors may tend to make men less responsive than women to the needs of a woman who self-injures. Esther, whose husband lacks empathy, has reached this conclusion on her own:

. . . .

I'm more comfortable having women see [my scars] than men. I think there is more sensitivity there. Most men don't seem to understand the depth of pain sometimes. I think they just don't get it. I mean, my husband has heard a lot of this stuff that I've been through and we talk about a lot of it, and he still says things like, "I just I don't get it, I don't *get* it! Why do you have to do it? Why do you have to go to therapy?" I think also that men see it as a weakness and I don't think that women see it that way as much.

. . . .

   The strains of partnership and parenthood can lead to tensions and explosive emotional reactions such as jealousy, frustration, and anger that feel as though they must be released through self-injury. Quarrels between partners can build anger that is diverted into self-cutting or -hitting, even in front of the partner. As Helena says concerning a quarrel with her lover, "I needed to hurt myself so bad I didn't care if he was there or not." Enraged with a lover, Erica once cut herself while in her lover's presence — the only time she has injured herself in front of anyone, and the only time she has cut herself in anger and frustration rather than to return from a state of dissociation. Even if the partner understands the need to self-injure, s/he may feel unfairly treated, fearing to be cross or critical again.
   In the following vignette, Karen tells how family life can encourage self-injury:

. . . .

I usually get up early and I start brooding right away about my situation, how trapped I feel and how anxious I feel. A typical day might start around four in the morning because I can't sleep. So I'll get up and read or something, or just brood. Sometimes I'll go for a walk in the dark. Then I come back and get ready for work and get the kids up. I go to work about nine o'clock.

My day consists of seeing elderly clients, doing reassessments, and having meetings. Most of the day, I keep pretty much to myself. I don't have any friends, really. I don't let people know how I feel basically, except my therapist, and sometimes my husband. And usually, by the end of the day I feel pretty down.

I always spend time running round, picking up my daughter at daycare, and transporting her back and forth. And that always makes me anxious because I feel as though everybody looks on me as a defective mother. I make use of a lot of community resources that are free or cheap, and I feel as though people look down on me. So, by the time I've seen a lot of these caregivers, I'm real anxious.

Then I go home, and the house is a *wreck* usually because my son has been there with his friends and they haven't been supervised after school because there's nobody there to supervise them. That makes me anxious and unhappy, and then I'm usually tense with my husband. Supper is usually awful and tense. The kids don't like what we serve so we have to make them a separate meal so they'll eat it. There's always teasing and loud behavior and I don't get any chance to talk to Jack [my husband], [or] to relax; there's no way to communicate about the day. After supper there's no time because Jack helps my son with his homework — there's just no *time*. By the time things are cleaned up and the kids are tucked away, and everything's over, it's about eleven o'clock at night and I'm all wound up.

Then, what usually happens is Jack and I have a fight or an argument about money because that's a real problem for us right now. We both are angry at each other, and I sit in silence and he reads — I mean, we're not talking, we're not communicating. I start to brood about it, and then I start to worry that I'll never get my life in order, and I'll never get things under control. I start to think about people in the past who have made me feel bad about myself — members of my family. And I count Jack in on that because he's done things to me that have undermined my confidence. The more I think about them, the angrier I get and the more unhappy I get. Then I just wait — I wait till he's asleep — and I want to be destructive with him. I don't do anything to *him* — but I end up cutting myself.

I go in the bathroom. I have a supply of razor blades, and I start cutting myself, just little places; then, after a while, I make a big slash, or two, or three — it depends. When it finally starts to hurt a little bit, I stop. Usually it doesn't hurt at first; I just don't feel it. If I make a really deep cut, I bandage it up real fast with tape so it won't make a horrendous mess. I don't want to look at it usually. Initially [I want to see it], and then I don't want to see it anymore for a while. Then I just sit for a while with myself and I feel a little better. I mean, I feel bad that I did it and I know there are going to be certain repercussions, but I feel relieved. I just sit for a while with myself, and then I go to bed.

· · · · · · · · · ·

Karen's two major concerns afflict many mothers who work within and outside the home: lack of time and money. There is not enough time for Karen to spend with her children, to talk to her husband, or to find even a few moments' peace. There is not enough money to enable her to buy more time through more extensive resources or fewer office hours. Her hectic day is spent caring for clients and children, with no opportunity to tell anyone how she feels. At home, voices raised in childish teasing or adult strife are followed by a brooding silence during which the day's tensions mix explosively with memories. Karen's accumulated anxiety, anger, and frustration lead to the one communication that always brings relief: self-injury.

On Mothers, Daughters, and Sons

Motherhood can raise complex questions for self-injuring women, beginning with the question of whether parenting is an appropriate option. Edith and Rosa say that they fear what they might do to their children should they have any. Edith specifically fears imitating her own mother and father: "I probably would have done some horrible things as a parent when I was younger, not knowing, and have repeated the pattern in some ways." Rosa's fears center around her father's behavior as well as her own: "As long as my father's alive, I don't want any possibility of my kids having anything to do with him." Rosa is also afraid that if she were a mother, she might physically assault her child in anger. Angry parents not considered abusive beat their children routinely under the euphemisms "spanking" or "discipline." Abused women, like Rosa, are perhaps more sensitive to any violation of a child's physical integrity, including socially condoned violations. Also, Rosa is sometimes tempted to pick at other people's scabs as well as her own: "I wouldn't want to do that to my kid." For Edith and Rosa, remaining childless is a preventive measure against perpetuating child abuse.

Prolonged abuse does seem to increase children's risk of growing up to abuse their own children, especially for men,[3] even though the great majority of adults who suffered childhood abuse do not abuse their own children.[4] One study suggests that emotional support from a nonabusive adult during childhood; past or present therapy; and a stable, nonabusive, emotionally sustaining relationship with a partner can help prevent an abused mother from abusing her children.[5] I did not ask my informants who are mothers whether they had ever abused their children. However, Karen volunteered that she sometimes felt like physically abusing her daughter when she was little, and at times was very close to doing so. Once she did abuse the child, and the Department of Social Services was called in: "It was an unbearable time. I had just gotten out of a four-month hospitalization. I felt utterly, utterly miserable. I have asked her to forgive me a thousand times. I've never hurt her since."

None of the mothers had felt deterred by self-injury in their decision to have children, perhaps partly because some of them were not injuring themselves during the time they conceived and bore children, or during the children's early years. However, almost half of the childless women say that self-injury will affect their decision to become mothers. They think that an environment in which self-injury occurs would be destructive for children and want to be free of self-injury before becoming mothers. Barbara, who because of childhood torture cannot give birth, would adopt a child but not unless she can stop cutting herself. She wants no child until she can be a "healthy role model," another way of expressing some women's wish to remain childless for fear of becoming abusers themselves or to help prevent their own children's exposure to self-injury. Sarah does not pinpoint self-injury but cites her refusal to pass on her genes as an argument against childbearing, another way of trying to prevent the continuation of emotional distress.

. . . .

I might consider adopting a child if I progress much more quickly than I am right now. I think I would like to have children but I would never until I'm certain that *I'm* grown up and that I can emotionally take care of myself and be available to take care of a child. There's tons of things that have to be considered when thinking about having a child, like what would I say if they asked me what the scars were from? How would I respond? Whether the child is my own or adopted, that will come up eventually, and I don't know how I would respond. But I would certainly never have a child of my own, and hopefully whatever genes are with me will die with me.

. . . .

Mothers do often find that self-injury affects their children's lives. Indeed, abused women's children may have to try to comprehend numerous disturbing aspects of their mothers' lives, including depression, dissociation, alter identities, suicide attempts, and self-injury. Because of this complex drama of a mother's life, self-injury may be only one of several concerns to a child and not the most important one.

Nonetheless, all the mothers I talked with revealed that self-injury by itself affected their children's lives. At the very least, fear of disrobing can restrict a mother's activities with her children:

. . . .

Karen: I don't want my kids to know. I don't know *how* I'd explain it to them. So, I wear clothes that cover me up. I never wear a bathing suit or wear short sleeves. That's the way I live. A lot of things that I might do, I can't do because of this. [If I didn't have to cut myself], I'd *use* my body and I'd feel good about it. I'd *do* things, you know, outdoor things where you can take your clothes off, and go swimming, and things like that. I just envision this freedom that I haven't had, especially with my kids, while they're little.

. . . .

Karen's words suggest some mothers' anguish at having to deprive themselves and their children of pleasurable activities together. Such deprivations are all the sadder by being, in the long-run, futile. Most children of the mothers I interviewed eventually saw their mothers' scars. Chance and the closeness of family life make disclosure hard to avoid over the years. Children see their mothers in the act of dressing or coming out of the shower, or a sleeve may slide up while cooking or driving, leading to critical moments for mother and child. Because of accidental disclosures and a mother's understandable reticence, several mothers say that they are not sure how much their children know.

Mothers' accidental or intentional disclosures and their children's reactions vary widely depending partly on the child's age, character, and sophistication.

Karen and Her Son, Age Twelve, and Daughter, Age Six

. . . .

My son doesn't ask about them; he doesn't like them. I have some scars on my wrist that he saw one time and he looked at them, then pulled my sleeve down to cover them up and turned away in dismay. I simply couldn't think of anything to say, so I didn't say anything. That was the only time I saw a real physical reaction from him. But the others I know he's seen. I've never said anything to him about them. I don't really know what he knows, to tell you the truth. It wasn't as though I could [tell a lie] as I would to a six-year-old. I'm sure he knew something then that he wasn't going to discuss with me. . . .

It's the most miserable feeling, knowing that something about you makes your child fearful and silent. My son did say once, "You're all scars, Mom; where'd you get cut so much?" and all I could say was, "Yeah, I know." I've never figured out a way to help him deal with it because he won't talk about it, even to a therapist. The one time we tried together it was a disaster. He has a hard time being affectionate with me now. I know he loves me, but it's from a distance.

. . . .

Karen, who told her daughter that she was "in an accident," knows that her son is too old to believe a lie. Yet the truth about the scars beneath her sleeve is too difficult to tell. She chooses silence, realizing that her son suspects or knows something and has also chosen silence.

Peggy and Her Son, Age Nine

. . . .

He recently told me that he knew. I had had another explosion and I went into the front hall and banged my head against the colonial column. He came into the room and I stood there with my hands over my eyes, and I was leaning against it. I think he had heard it. Then we had to go pick up the babysitter. I asked him, straight out, about what he had understood that had happened. And I talked about how I got really angry, and that it was something that wasn't his fault, and what did he notice about my getting angry. He told me, "Well, I heard you when I came in and I saw your head there and I knew that you had banged it." I asked him how he knew that. . . . He said, "I've seen you before when you thought I wasn't looking." So, he knew.

I feel really bad in a way, because I don't know how long he had been sitting on that without telling anybody about it. We talked about it a little bit and I haven't brought it up again, but I feel like I need to. . . . I'm not quite sure what to do about it or how to handle it. It's pretty upsetting because I feel like it must be affecting him. I don't want him to go to school and tell his friends about it. I even told him that. I said, "I hope you're not going to just talk to anybody about that. But I also don't want you to think that you can never talk about it. If you need to talk about it, maybe we could figure out who you could talk to about it." I'm embarrassed by it, and I'm trying to explain that to him: "*You* don't need to be ashamed of this; it's me who feels that way." It's hard because I have to figure out a way to help him to deal with it, because I don't want him to grow up messed up.

He also said that he'd seen me kick the wall and punch the wall, that sort of thing. I think I realized he'd seen that. I feel a little freer sometimes hitting the wall or kicking the wall, or kicking the cabinets.

When I'm like that, he tries to take care of me. He asks me if I need a hug, because he knows that I love hugs. He kind of stays away—he gets cautious. He keeps a distance, but he tries to look and you can tell that his little brain is figuring out what to do. He asks me if I need a hug, but he stays far enough back so that if I'm not quite over being angry, or whatever, he is not in the way. He is really cautious about what to do but he also tries to be there. He almost seems to put himself in the line of fire in a way just in case I want a hug. And I talk to him about that. I said, "I'm the mom, I'm the grownup, I'm the one who's supposed to teach you how to deal with anger, and I'm the one who's supposed to take care of you when you are feeling bad. It bothers me that you feel like you need to take care of me when I'm feeling bad."

. . . .

Peggy's experience tells of myriad subtle emotions. She feels guilt and anguish upon discovering that her son knows about her self-injury and has had to live with this knowledge alone. She is simultaneously fearful that he will indiscriminately reveal her secret and, conversely, that he will feel unable to talk about it at all. Most of all, she does not want him to suffer during childhood as she did, or to feel that he has to take care of her. When faced with a crisis in his mother's behavior, Peggy's son acts like a wise adult. He does not cry, sulk, whine, or retreat. Instead, he blends love and strategy by assessing the situation, comforting her and himself with signs of affection, yet protecting himself from possible harm.

Mary and Her Daughters, Ages Nineteen and Twenty-two

. . . .

My youngest one lives with me, and I don't wear long sleeves twenty-four hours a day. I don't wear them all the time anyway; it depends on who I'm with. She can see them; it's that simple. She knew what they were. When she asked me, [I told her]. She was eighteen. She said, "What are you cutting yourself with?" She asked me what it felt like and I told her; and she asked me if I thought I could stop, and I said I was really trying to work on it. I tried to be as honest as I could, and I said, "I can't tell you I'm not going to anymore. I would love to be able to do that for myself." We had some conversations on it. I felt that it would be better for her to be honest about it, and so we've talked about it quite a bit. She told me about a girl she's working with right now who doesn't just cut, she actually cuts words into her skin. . . .

To tell you the truth, by then, she knew about so many other things that it was like one more thing. I haven't gone into detail, but I told her about my background. She knows about the multiple personality disorder—both of [my daughters] do. She has been to a session with me with a social worker at a hospital and also with my psychiatrist where she has had an opportunity to ask a lot of questions so that she can become somewhat knowledgeable. I think that has been really good.

. . . .

Mary bears scars from childhood torture as well as from self-cutting, but many of them are well faded with age. She does not feel the same degree of shame about them as many women do. Her younger daughter is a sophisticated young adult, already knowledgeable about cutting. This combination allows an honest discussion about self-injury. Mary's daughter is, understandably, concerned about her mother, even more so since the time that Mary cut a vein and had to be hospitalized.

Signs of childhood trauma have brought the younger daughter closer to Mary, but they have alienated the older daughter. Although the older daughter is also knowledgeable, through schoolmates and colleagues, about self-injury, there are no frank discussions about it between her and her mother. Age and knowledge about cutting do not prevent Mary's older daughter from temporarily rejecting Mary, whom the daughter always saw only as a "superwoman" parent and successful worker, and now has trouble accepting as anything else.

Esther and Her Daughter, Age Seventeen, and Son, Age Nineteen

. . . .

When it comes to talking about anything, she doesn't really want to know, so I don't give her much information. She asked me a long time ago why I started going into therapy and I said, "Let's go out for breakfast and we'll talk about it." She was twelve and I thought she was old enough to understand about what rape is and things like that. So I started off the conversation by just saying that I had been raped when I was a child. And she said, "Who was the bastard?" And when I told her it was her grandfather she said, "You mean *Dad's* dad?" And I said, "No, not Dad's dad; *my* father." And she goes, "Oh, that's so *sick!*" But there were no questions; she was taking this as fact. And I said, "It is a very difficult thing and I don't expect you to understand some of the things that you might see, but I thought you should know exactly what's going on." She was fine with that. She didn't ask me any questions. It was just like, "Okay, that's all I need to know."

As far as self-injury goes, she really doesn't know much about that part of me at all. She has seen some scars. I had a scar here on my wrist and she asked me about that. She thought that I had tried to kill myself. And I said, "No, I wasn't really intending to cut there; I had intended to cut further up my arm. But I didn't have much control and I cut my wrist instead of further up my arm." And she said, "What do you mean you were trying to cut your arm?" I said, "I can't explain why." At that point, I really didn't understand it much myself. And she said, "So this is just stuff that you have to go through?" And I said, "Well, it's stuff that I go through; I don't know if it's stuff I *have* to go through, so don't think it's required that you cut yourself in order to heal from incest. It's just one of my ways of coping." She kind of took that and, "Oh, okay." It didn't really bother her too much after that as long as it didn't look like I was doing any deep damage.

. . . .

Esther's daughter seems to have a matter-of-fact attitude to her mother's self-injury and to accept it as being "stuff that you have to go through" if you were raped by your father. She can tell the difference between the cutting that her mother does and suicide attempts, and appears not to be concerned about Esther's physical safety.

Esther's son sees things differently. He, too, knows about the self-injury:

. . . .

One time my son noticed a lot of cuts on my arm. He asked me about it, and I said, "Oh that's nothing; don't worry about it." And he grabbed my hand and he goes, "It's *nothing?* Take a look at that, Mom, it's something. What happened? Did the cat scratch you?" And I said, "No, the cat didn't scratch me. I just got a little carried away with my knife." That was the first time he realized what I meant by hurting myself.

. . . .

Esther's son now has subtle ways of taking care of her, probably not only because of the cutting but because he knows that she has periods of depression and dissociation and has tried to die. In the evening, if he notices that Esther is depressed or "not quite there," he spends time with her before he goes out to make sure that she is alright. He will sit with her in the livingroom and talk with her or join in what she is doing: putting together a puzzle, watching television. Although neither mother nor son explicitly acknowledges his reasons for being there, a number of times on such evenings Esther has said, "It's okay, you can go now. I'm fine."

Jessica and Her Son, Age Seventeen, and Daughter, Age Twenty
. . . .
I don't remember a real finding out, but I have taken them swimming. As best I could I've tried to keep [the acts themselves] from them, but they've seen the scars. There's so much in my life that they don't want to know about, and the scars and the self-injury are just in that package. I don't really know how much they know; we haven't gone into that. It was during a period when they were actually interested in knowing [which alter identity] was up and trying to figure out who was who and what they could get out of them. . . . So, self-abuse and scars got in there with trying to figure out "Who do I tell about this?" and the suicidality. If there was much asking back and forth it was more in terms of, "Oh, that's yet another thing to add to your stack of 'Mummy's weird, and you don't really want to know.'"
. . . .

Both of Jessica's children are in therapy, and Jessica tells her own and her children's therapists all they might need to know to help her children. Jessica has "passing conversations" with her children about trauma, multiple identities, and self-injury. About self-injury she tells them, "This is what I do. It has nothing to do with you. It is because of all that happened to me."

As these vignettes suggest, effects of childhood trauma can spill over into the next generation. A mother's self-injury appears to leave a legacy for her children. Some children may grow into adults who have a compassionate understanding of self-injury and other emotional distresses. However, this compassion may be gained at a price of strained bonds between mother and child through secrecy, silence, or the perceived need to take care of a mother. Mothers have the added strain of trying to know how best to explain self-injury to a child, and weighing the benefits and awkwardness of silence against the difficulties of openness. As mothers, they are attempting to protect their children from emotional harm while living with the severe consequences of their own damaged childhoods.

Friendships

. . . .
Elizabeth: There's just one circle of friends where we're all really close, and they know. We've all been sexually abused, and it was really *that* that brought us together. They're my best friends now. But other friends don't know; it's just that one small group. And one night I was cutting, and one of my friends

called. She knew that I had just cut, and she just started crying. She was crying hysterically saying, "I don't want you to die. We don't want to lose you; we're going to lose you." Only two days before I had been talking to my counselor and I said, "I don't see what the harm in doing this is, because it doesn't affect anybody else, only me." And she said, "Don't you think it affects your friends, or me, or your family?" I said, "No." And then, all of sudden, my friend was calling me and she was crying on the phone.

They relate it to other things that we all deal with. . . . But I know that cutting is only one symptom of the problem, and the problem is sexual abuse. My friends have gone to other things to deal with it like sex- and love-addiction, alcoholism, eating disorders. So, when they relate it to sexual abuse they understand, but when they look at the cutting, *my* symptom, they don't understand.

My friends sometimes get angry because I didn't go to them first before I cut; I just went ahead and cut. When I was in Albany my very best friend was like, "Let's go out and buy some watermelon, and I'll go get some bubble bath so you can have a hot bath, and we'll talk." I was like, "Okay." And she said, "Alright, so you won't cut while I go out to the store," and I said, "No." But I knew I would; I just wanted to get rid of her. I'm not at that point yet where I'm willing to take it a step further and say, "No, don't leave, because if you leave, I will cut." I'm not there yet, and I let her leave. As soon as she walked out the door, I did it. I told her later on that night that I had done it, and she was very upset, because she said, "You know, I really thought it would make you feel better if I tried to do all those things for you. I just feel so helpless because I don't think there is anything I can do." That gets hard. Because then, I got angry, and I kept saying, "Well, I shouldn't have told you, then." I guess it's good and bad, in a way, [for my best friends to know]. People from the outside would say it's all good, but I would say it's good and bad.

[Even with this close circle of friends] I don't tell them every time I do it. I rarely tell them. I'll just call them up after not talking to them for a week or so, and they'll say something like, "So how's the cutting going?" And I'll say, "Oh, don't ask." I won't say, "Well, I cut last night, and I cut the night before and I cut the night before that." I don't like to get into specifics because I don't like to draw attention to it. So I'll just tell them the general: "Yes, it's still going on; but don't ask me any more than that."

If I cut, I won't call my friends for days. As soon as I cut, I'm back into the isolation again and I want the world to leave me alone and I don't want to be a part of it. When I cut on myself, it cuts me off from everyone. I know [it's partly because of] shame, especially with me and my friends where we have open, honest friendships, and we know absolutely everything about each other. My friends would sometimes ask me about my progress, and I can't lie to them, but I don't want them to know. So I think that it's just easier for me to — not call! I haven't called my best friend in quite a while. She's left messages on my machine and I won't return her calls. Sometimes it seems like it's easier to not have to worry about what anyone's going to think. It's me — my thing — and the fewer people that know the better; the fewer people that get involved, the better. I have to [sometimes lie to my friends] because if they knew the amount of times that I did it, they would be more worried than they should be. I would rather lie than have them overreact.

[Also,] my two roommates asked me quite a few times what happened to my arm. Of course I made up a story because I couldn't tell them the truth. And even though the subject was dropped after that point, I still can't go around and show the scars. Today, I had to leave work early and my roommates were not at home when I got home. It was so great; it was almost like a treat that I was able to go in with no sweater on and wear a sleeveless shirt. I felt free. It might sound trivial, but it really felt good. Even though they have dropped the subject and they won't ask me again, I still can't do it. They're there and they're looking at the scars, and my roommates are people who are a part of my life. I don't care if a total stranger sees my scars.

But with my close friend and her husband, they both know, and they're really understanding about it. It's so nice to be able to walk into their house and take off my sweater. They don't react. They know the scars are there, but they act like they're totally oblivious to them. They don't look at them, they don't mention them, they don't comment on them. They don't say, "God, they look *awful!*" And it's really good because I don't have to worry about it then. I know that I can walk into their house and not worry about defending myself, or feeling guilty or ashamed. It makes a difference; it's great. It's almost like I'm walking into neutral ground. You know, I almost feel like I'm on a battlefield sometimes, and I feel like it's me against the whole world. Sometimes I feel like I'm on the outside looking in. I don't even feel like I *belong*. And it's so nice to just go into neutral ground where I don't feel that.

· · · · · · · · · ·

As long as only self-injury can give Elizabeth the solace and release she needs, it takes precedence even over the closest friendship. A friend will naturally want to keep her from what is perceived as self-harm. Therefore, complete honesty with friends is undesirable: Elizabeth's primary allegiance is to self-injury, her greatest "friend."

As Elizabeth's account also suggests, because self-injury is such an engrossing and secret part of a woman's life, it can define friendship: a close friend is a person one trusts enough to tell about self-injury. There are other types of friends, ones who want to hear that you are fine and feel well—nothing else; friends with whom one goes out to dinner once in a while or to the movies or theater. These are friends strictly for diversion, entertainment, and general social life, and they may serve these important functions well. Nonetheless, they are not necessarily people whom one entrusts with a secret.

Choosing the select few for disclosure about self-injury may be a simple matter: some women who self-injure disclose only to other self-injurers or, at the most, to other women who experienced incest or other severe abuses during childhood. These confidants are the ones whose backgrounds are similar, the ones who know the power of overwhelming emotions, the ones who can understand the need to self-injure. One can have fun with them, but also sit and talk about living with self-injury without worrying about repulsion or rejection:

. . . .

Jane: I have friends who have harmed themselves, and it's something we understand in each other. We don't condemn one another for it, but if we're talking and one of us is thinking of doing it, we can sometimes talk one another out of it. But there's no condemnation. Because you know you're talking to somebody who's done it, you don't have the level of shame or embarrassment. Sometimes, we can even joke about it—it sounds morbid to other people—little things, like, "Well, I don't go as deep as you do," or "I don't make them as long as you do." Or [we sometimes joke about] what we can wear. It depends on the mood. Part of it is that we can support each other and help each other not do it. Other people, they really don't understand it. Just having them find out is embarrassing.
. . . .

Making and keeping close friends can take time and care for anyone. This can be especially true for a person who has a problem generally considered taboo. Edith is a woman who has worked at having good friends who have no connection to mental health problems or psychiatric hospitals. Through her professional life and hobbies, she has a group of friends who know about her childhood abuse and even about her alter identities. They "can handle" the fact that she has multiple identities and sometimes joke about it in ways that do not offend her. She considers herself a good judge of character and feels fortunate that she has had such positive responses from her friends. But about self-injury?

. . . .

Edith: Very few people know about that, and even the people who "know," know it only in the abstract. I've never really gone into it. I mean, it was hard enough to even say that picking at things is a problem. I have not gone into detail at all because I just figured that this was too much. . . . It's like, "Oh God, no, that's too gross. Everybody would think I'm just—*yuck.*" That's been the biggest secret of all.

. . . .

Like other women who self-injure, Edith carefully chooses whom to tell. When she does decide to disclose this ultimate secret, she doesn't say, "I *gouge* at my skin." She chooses her words carefully: "You know how you always see scratches and band-aids on me? Well, that's one of the problems that I have because I'm always scratching away at scabs and making things bleed." With every word, she watches her listener's face for signs of disgust. She stops talking as soon as she perceives that her listener has had enough.

Despite Edith's care in making friends outside the mental health system and despite her fondness for these friends, her relief is obvious when she describes talking with women who injure themselves:

. . . .

It's incredible for me to sit there and have somebody talk about it and describe many of the same feelings that I'm feeling, or the conflicts. There are a lot of differences between how we feel, or what we do, but it's just incredible to have somebody understand in here [points to her heart] what I'm saying as opposed to somebody like you or my therapist who's never *done* this, who can't understand at that level. Theoretically, you can understand it; but you don't get it at the gut level. And that's what's been so helpful for me. For them to say, "Oh, I know what you mean" when I'm talking, or for me to say, "Yes, that's exactly how I feel" when they're talking is very affirming. It's not that it makes it alright, but somehow having somebody who knows to share it with makes it better and makes me not so much of an isolate.

. . . .

Edith is one of four women who were self-injuring at the time of their disclosure but had positive responses after confiding in friends who neither self-injured nor had experienced childhood abuse. These four women—Edith, Erica, Barbara, and Mary—are among those who have found trustworthy companions, often people who have shared heartaches and celebrations for years, and whose intimacy includes personal struggles of all kinds. Some women's friendships have become closer as a result of confiding about self-injury. These women have found that even when friends feel helpless or un-comfortable about self-injury, they can be understanding, encouraging, and comforting.

Correct choice of a confidant is crucial, and not every woman is fortunate. One rejection after disclosure can discourage all further attempts. Karen is one who was mistreated by a friend after confiding in her: "She just pulled back and didn't say why, . . . and that was that." This friend also implied that Karen was a potential danger to the friend's child. This experience confirmed Karen's opinion that "no one understands it really, and it scares people." As to her other friends, Karen feels that she lacks the energy to try to explain self-injury to them. Instead of bringing Karen closer to selected friends, disclosure seems to feed her sense of isolation:

· · · · · · · · ·

I feel different, and strange, and I feel *obsessed* by it, and I'd give anything to get rid of the obsession. I'd give anything to put the razor blades in the back-ground — not think about them anymore, not have them be an answer to feeling bad. But, I can't give it *up*! I feel really different from other people as a result, and lonely, real lonely.

· · · · · · · · ·

Because secrecy can prevail between people who think they know each other well, strange situations may arise. Peggy usually finds self-injury a barrier to getting closer to her friends with whom she discusses depression, medica-tions, and therapy, but not self-injury. However, in the course of one con-versation about depression, Judy — Peggy's friend of four years — suddenly said that as a child she had banged her head against the wall. Peggy replied, "Judy, you don't know who you're talking to." Thus began a process of confidences that deepened the two women's friendship by transforming self-injury from a barrier into a bridge.

Erica sees self-injury as a part of her that her friends do not even know exists: "To me it's like this fundamental piece of information because it's such a presence in my life and they don't know about it." A painful situation with friends arose because of that vital missing piece, with Erica and her partner the silent victims of one friend's insensitivity:

· · · · · · · · ·

There was one very awkward time I can think of. We were out having lunch with some friends and one of them is a clinical social worker. She was going on and on about something and she said, "Oh yeah, and then we had some-body come in to talk to us about the slice-and-dicers." And I was sitting there going, "I can't look up. I have to just sit here and move my food around the plate." She went on a few more minutes about them, and neither one of us responded to anything she was saying, and [that] finally just stopped the topic. But I just sat there looking at my plate the whole time. So that comes to mind as just how wide the chasm was: she was sitting there across the table thinking that she was joking with people who shared this perspective when in fact, the people across the table from her were being impacted by it in a very different way. That was a dreadful moment.

. . . .

Friends who do not know the secret are those whose reactions to the truth could be painful. The essence of the fears are these words: "They will see me differently and turn away." These fears sound familiar to anyone who has done something s/he is unwilling to tell a friend or partner. Fear of disclosure can vary depending on the degree of social unacceptability of the self-injury involved. A woman who bites her fingers and picks at acne may be less concerned because she knows that many people bite their nails and cuticles, sometimes to the point of rawness and bleeding, or pick at sores and scabs. Greater fear may be attached to head- or limb-banging, and the greatest fear of all to self-cutting. Rejection during adulthood can cause severe emotional problems even for those whose childhood relationships were safe and secure. Women already so severely betrayed by caregivers in their younger years are especially likely to want to avoid as adults the risk of rejection that disclosure can bring:

. . . .

Karen: They might respond sympathetically, but then they might pull back, thinking, "I don't understand this kind of thing; it scares me, so I'm going to pull back." Because I've told people before and then I've sensed the pulling back even though there was no particular reason for it: we were still friendly. And I thought, "Well, maybe it was that they just didn't know what to say and it was unnerving to them." So, I don't know. I tell almost no one. In fact, even my sister who I'm really close to, I never talk to her about it, never. I just don't want to turn people off, and I think that would be the result. They wouldn't get it; they wouldn't see why somebody would need to do that.

. . . .

Even other women who endured childhood incest but do not self-injure may not understand, and could say something hurtful. Esther had such an experience when someone from her discussion group for sexually-abused women said, "I saw a thing on television about that, and they said that people do that for attention. Do you think that you do that for attention?" This painful mis-conception stayed with Esther, who now fears that other friends might think that "Esther is just looking for attention." As Esther says, "I think that if someone wants attention there are a lot of better ways to get [it]; a lot of bet-ter ways. . . ."

Because of their past experiences, some self-injuring women find that they have to train themselves to allow a person to be an intimate friend. Having had their trust and love grotesquely violated as children, they may understand-ably be reluctant to trust or grow fond of anyone again. In her teens and twen-ties, Barbara had a policy of never getting close to people: "I wanted it to be that anyone in my life could die at any moment and I wouldn't shed a tear because it wouldn't matter. That was what safety felt like to me." Barbara even-tually realized that her self-imposed isolation and disconnection were intoler-able. During the past ten years she has allowed emotional attachments back into her life and gradually gathered a circle of intimate friends.

Now, when necessary, Barbara also instructs her friends. A friend in whom a self-injuring woman wishes to confide is ideally prepared for confidence if she too self-injures. She is likely to be prepared if she suffers from sex-, food-, or drug-addiction related to childhood abuse, although even here it may be hard for a person to imagine that self-injury can be as addictive or appealing as food, alcohol, or other mind-altering substances. She is somewhat prepared if her child self-injures. She has a slight advantage if she has suffered from other embarrassing signs of emotional distress such as hair-pulling, compul-sive counting or washing, or irrational fears. In all these examples, a friend's own experiences have given her (or him) at least a basic idea of why a woman would need to injure herself.

What can be done if a trustworthy friend has had no such experiences? Barbara has found a way of using analogy to help a friend understand and respond with empathy to self-injury:

. . . .

My friendships are very intimate. We know everything about each other's lives. If I feel like cutting, I call up my friends and talk about it. I have some friends that are recovering cutters themselves. But I also have friends who would never even think of cutting themselves, but they understand that that is part of who I am and they accept it and try to help me if I ask for it. Some aren't recovering alcoholics or anything like that, and some come from func-tional—whatever a functional family is. But mostly, in my circle of closest friends, Jenny is an incest survivor, so she knows. Carol has never been an alcoholic but she struggles with food addiction. She's not grossly overweight, but she knows what it is like to have to . . . go out and buy cookies in the middle of the night. She can imagine the compulsion. My friend Susan doesn't have a clue [as] to what addiction is about; she's not addicted to anything. I have to explain it to her. . . . She likes to eat but she's not even compulsive about that. She likes to drink water. If she's thirsty, she'll drink. I say, "Can you imagine if you were in the desert for weeks and weeks without any water and you know you are barely living, and finally you get to water and the people that have the water want to have a conversation before they give it to you? All you're thinking about is, 'Give me the goddamn water!' Your whole mind, every part of your body is saying, 'I want a drink, I want a drink.'" . . . I say, "That's what it feels like to be addicted. To have something screaming out, whether it's my razor blades: 'Oh, I need to cut, I need to cut, I need to cut.' Or whether it's: 'I want a drink' or 'I want a drug' or 'I want a cookie.'" She has never been there herself but she is sympathetic. You can have empathy without having had to live it, but usually you have to have a similar something that you can translate into that. That water analogy worked for her. She gets it.

. . . .

Women who self-injure have to teach others how to respond to self-injury in ways that are helpful and painless — not always an easy task. One way of learning is to listen to women as they tell how, ideally, they would want a friend to respond:

. . . .

Jane: Don't panic, get angry, or condemn me. Talk compassionately with me. If I have just cut, help me assess whether or not I need stitches, but without making me feel bad about myself whatever I decide to do.

. . .

Edith: Say to me, "Oh, I'm *sorry* you felt you had to do that. It must hurt a lot inside for you to do that." Acknowledge the pain that self-injury represents.

. . .

Karen: Don't say that I'm "sick" and need to go to the hospital. That just makes me feel more isolated and weird. Tell me that you're sorry that I feel so bad, but that you can support me and remain my friend. Embrace me and say, "I can see why you want to do this."

. . .

Elizabeth: I want you to ignore my scars and never ask me about them so that I won't have to explain them to you. I know, though, that ideally I should be telling you each time I cut so that I'd feel ashamed and perhaps do it less.

. . .

Erica: Depending on my mood, I may want you to be sympathetic and say, "Oh, that must be very hard for you." But if I'm being defensive about it, I just want you to say, "Oh, okay," and leave me alone (although I realize that just dismissing it may be too much to ask from someone who does not self-injure).

. . .

Peggy: Show me acceptance, understanding, and *some* concern, not too much. Don't just dismiss it either. Perhaps ask me a question about it; say that I could talk with you about it if I want to.

. . .

Jessica: Acknowledge the pain I'm in. See this as a way that I'm expressing my emotions, like crying.

. . .

Barbara: Don't react as though this were something you could catch. Be somewhat concerned or interested but not overly dramatic about it. Perhaps ask me, "Are you getting help for it?"

. . .

Rosa: Don't make me feel like a freak, or ashamed, or sick. Show me that you're concerned. Ask me if I'm dealing with it and how. Say that I could talk with you about it if I want to, but that I don't have to. Praise me for working on this with my therapist.

. . .

Esther: Don't give me a hug; I don't want a physical response. Show me that you're concerned, not for the injuries themselves but for what's behind them.

. . .

Sarah: Don't ask me about my scars because I either have to lie or tell the truth, neither of which I want to do. If you care and are trying to reach out and be my friend, let me know in other ways that I can talk with you about it if I need to.

. . .

Helena: I feel so conflicted about it myself that it's hard to know how I want someone to react. Don't think I'm nuts, don't pity me, and don't think self-injury is "cool." Take it in stride; that would be exactly right.

. . .

Caroline: Just listen in a nonjudgmental way; don't make us more separate. We're all human.

. . .

Meredith: I want you to ask me the questions you're wondering about because if you don't ask, you won't understand self-injury any better. But, I want you to ask because you want to understand, not because you think I'm a freak.

• • •

Mary: React the way you would if I told you I had breast cancer and had to have a mastectomy. It's an uncomfortable thing to talk about, but acceptable. Treat this like a physical illness and help make it acceptable.

• • • • • • • • • •

In sum, most of these women want acknowledgment, compassion, and some concern for the feelings that underlie self-injury. They welcome reassurance that the friendship can remain intact, and that they need not fear anger, condemnation, or rejection. They want to be able to talk about self injury, if they wish, and find an interested, understanding, and nonjudgmental ear.

Partners, family members, and friends may want to remind themselves not to take self-injury personally, or to set ultimatums for stopping. Both of these responses can be damaging to the self-injuring woman and to the relationship with her. Remember that any positive relationship is itself a sign of success in overcoming an abused woman's past. It is laudable that self-injuring women attempt and successfully manage friendships, partnerships, and motherhood. Self-injury, itself a way of coping with prior destructive relationships, should not be allowed to disrupt current healthy ones.

6 Helena's Struggle With Compulsion

WHEN I WAS growing up, I always thought I was nuts! I thought that nobody else in the whole world was doing this except for me. . . . I know how I felt in the [abuse survivor] group when I admitted that I did this, and the facilitator said, "Who else does that?" Everybody, *everybody* did. And I said, "Wow! I never knew anybody who said that they did this. . . ." There could have been people who did it and weren't telling me; *I* certainly wasn't telling anybody. So, I [had] thought: "Oh this is just another thing about me that proves I'm crazy."

I was not actively [injuring myself in grade school] but when I think about it, I used to do things like put the desk in front of me on my foot, and when the kid came back and sat down it would be very painful, but I would transcend it. So I used to do things like that, sort of active/passive ways of hurting myself. I used to love to get shots. When I went to the doctor, I always wanted a shot — [well,] not always, there was a time when I hated shots. . . . [But from] a certain point [in my life], I liked shots. I was like, "Am I going to get a shot this time?" I've always been proud of my high pain threshold. . . . I was dissociating, I think. But also my mother has a very low pain threshold, and it's possible that I was trying to separate myself from her.

When I was in high school, my hair was [down to the] middle of my back. After college, basically right before I started remembering [and] dealing with the fact that there was some kind of abuse going on, I cut off my hair to under my ears. And then that summer I cut it all the way off so that it was like a little pixie cut. And it got shorter and shorter till it was like a crewcut it was so short. I stopped going to the hairdresser [and] used to cut it myself. I told myself it was to save money, but I would often cut off my hair when I was upset with myself and wanted to hurt myself. I would wildly attack my head with the scissors and sometimes I would accidentally — I wasn't intending to, but it was a consequence that I would accidentally cut myself in the back of the neck. I would have huge bald spots and would have to have friends come and fix my hair. It was something of a statement because I was young. I wasn't wearing a bra, I was very radical, and my hair [was] another way of expressing my identity. But also I used it to attack myself, to make myself look a little strange. . . .

In high school I used to carry around in my purse the top of a wire hanger that I had twisted off. And when I would get upset with myself at school, I would say, "Excuse me . . . I have to go to the bathroom." I would go to the bathroom and cut myself. But I would do it [in] such a way that I could do it as much as I wanted and it would be very painful but I wouldn't bleed until later. It would be a scratch that bleeds only after it crusts over. Later, I would pick off the scabs and then I would bleed. . . . I like to see myself bleed. You know, I pick off scabs and I like to watch; it's the same kind of thing. And I used to keep my nails very, very short. That was a protective measure *and* a self-injurious thing because I sometimes cut them too far down. So I wouldn't scratch myself but I would get self-injury in by cutting them too short. But now they are about an eighth of an inch long. I try to keep them nice and I don't scratch myself.

If it looked obviously like I had done it myself then I might wear long sleeves. I remember one time I scraped a lot of the skin off of my forearm. It had huge scabs [but] it wasn't obvious that I had done it myself; it looked random. And a friend said, "Ooh! What did you do?" I said, "An accident." I certainly didn't tell anyone; I didn't advertise that I was doing this, but I didn't necessarily also make sure no one could see that I was injured. In fact, I felt proud of it; I felt good about it. It was like a battle scar: [it] proved [that I had been] grievously wounded and survived. [When I hid my scars, I did so because] I didn't want anyone to think I was a basket case or a mental case and to look down on me or to pity me or to stop hanging out with me — leave me because they couldn't handle me. . . .

You know, I don't want to see myself as being the product of certain things that happened when I was a child and that's it. I am trying very hard lately not to attribute everything to that. But having said all that, I don't remember if I mentioned to you that I am a sexual abuse survivor. . . . The sexual abuse started when I was about three and lasted till I was around eleven. Two of the perpetrators were extended family members: my uncle and my grandfather, but from opposite sides of the family. The other person was a family friend. And then I had some incidents as a teenager and in my early twenties [of] abusive relationships. I repressed my abuse for years and was injuring myself in high school before I remembered about the abuse. . . . So, in my mind it's linked but not linked. But I do wonder if I would self-injure in the same way if I hadn't had the history. I mean, it definitely colored my entire development. I'm hedging this way because I don't want everything to be attributed to those events in my life. It is not the only bad thing that ever happened, and I don't want people to be able to write it off that way, or write *me* off that way — that I am solely a product of this *thing* that happened.

I live in a sexist culture; there are a lot of reasons out there for me to feel bad about myself. I think women in mainstream American culture have self-loathing and conflicted relationships with their own bodies. I know that I do. I think it's not just from things that happened in childhood, although I think it certainly contributed. I think that it has to do equally with the whole culture and the messages that we get, and family messages are also part of the culture. So, I try to diversify my identity. . . .

Maybe in my case . . . I [took] up cutting myself as opposed to alcohol or drugs [because] . . . it had something to do with feeling like "Why can't anybody *see*," even though I largely repressed the stuff that was going on. I have some memories of trying to get my mother's attention, trying to tell my mother something's wrong, although I wasn't consciously thinking this way. It was the early '70s; she had no idea, she didn't pick up on this at all — which is not her fault. . . .

When I was in the fifth grade I asked my mom, "Can I see a psychologist?" I asked her . . . because I had read a book in which the main character had a lot of problems, and went to see a psychologist, and felt better. I knew that I had a lot of problems and I felt really bad about myself. And I said [to myself], "Well, I can do what this character in this book did." Little did I know that my friend down the street had just started seeing a therapist. *I* didn't know this . . . but my mother thought I wanted to be just like her, so it took me trying to cut my wrists when I was in the fifth grade for my mother to finally take me. I did it practically in order for my mother to see it, but I did it because I was tormented. It happens to have coincided with one of the major times that my grandfather abused me, one of the times that he had me alone — although my mother didn't know that. And my mom was like, "Okay, now we'll go see a therapist." I went maybe three or four months, and I don't even remember why I stopped going. But this therapist never asked me [about] sexual abuse. This was 1979. Who knew?

I don't mind talking about [what brought the memories back] but it certainly is different for everybody and for me it was gradual, with flashes of things and eventually piecing things together. I have incomplete memories where I'm pretty sure that I was in such and such a place with such and such a person, but the memories come in fragments. The first memory that I had was about the family friend: it was like it was all dark and I could see this one tiny dot with two people in it. I barely could tell who they were. In the memory I got closer and closer and closer and closer to it and then I saw that it was me and this man. But it was very much outside myself. All the memories come as, "Oh, that poor little girl" — looking at something happening to this figure who is me, as opposed to a memory where I would be inside looking out at something happening to me.

Sometimes there is movement and so it would be like an old nickelodeon — but that's just the visual memories. There are other memories that I'll have that don't have visuals, or I will have a visual memory and then other memories will come and attach to it, such as how old I feel in the memory; body memories — feeling the physical sensations; or emotional memories where I get very upset and I'm not exactly sure what to attach it to. I'm trying to work on recovering the emotional pieces because I'll have visual memory and can hear things happening and can feel them but don't have the emotions that were attached. And every time I get close to them it's so terrifying that I lose it.

I would say that most of the time I feel dissociated . . . to a greater or lesser extent. . . . Since the abuse started when I was so young and I dissociated it at that point, I don't know if I know what it's like not to be dissociated. So, if I weren't, I don't know if I would recognize it. It is so hard to figure out if this is my normal state.

It is really hard to describe dissociation; and it runs on a continuum. [When] there's a least amount of dissociation, I just feel like I'm outside of myself, like my life is a movie and I'm acting in my life and I'm doing things [and] things are happening to my body but it isn't *me* somehow. I'm not sure who I think I am but everything seems unreal: I feel removed from it. And yet I continue to go out and be an agent in the world. I do things certainly: I make things happen for myself, and it's not that I have no sense of the consequences of my actions; I just feel like it isn't me. I have actually regressed and acted like a little bitty child and been somehow aware that I was not four or five, but feeling completely other from my grown-up self. . . . That happens infrequently, but this feeling of being removed is pretty constant. I don't know what it would feel like not to feel this way, so sometimes I suspect that everybody feels this way and that I am giving myself this problem that everybody must have. But I don't know.

I think it's different [from daydreaming] because it's not that my thoughts are going far away. When I'm dissociated, I'm not necessarily distracted. . . . It is different from when I am lost in thought because right now I'm talking to you, I'm not lost in thought somewhere else, I'm not distracted, but I have a feeling that this isn't really happening. It feels like it's happening to someone else. It's more of a sense of being inside myself looking out through eyes that aren't mine. It's like everything is unreal. It's a numbing out, even if nothing is really happening, if I'm just eating breakfast or something. My therapist [used to say], "Touch something — touch the texture of something, put your feet on the floor, ground yourself." These things sometimes help but usually it doesn't really help.

[I'm twenty-eight now, and] I still have a lot of compulsions to self-injure but I just don't do it any more in the same way. I used to hit myself and cut myself [because] I was trying to get equilibrium from two extremes: either I was so upset that I had to cut myself to relieve it, or I was so numb that I had to cut myself to get back to being there. I would [also] hit myself with a big stick that I used to keep, [or] pound myself or pound the walls so I would get black and blue on my hand. I would be very angry or frustrated with myself. A lot of it is perfectionism; I'm a procrastinating perfectionist, so it's really bad: I don't give myself time to do a good job. When I was in school if I wasn't getting my work done it might happen, or if I felt myself to be failing in another way, [or] having done something stupid.

I no longer do the active thing, [but] I suspect that I have carried the behavior over and channeled it into other behaviors. When I feel depressed or angry with myself or numb or in a great deal of pain, I do other things that are more passive but I think are self-injurious. So, I no longer take knives and cut myself or take sticks and beat myself. . . . Now if I'm feeling those same ways, I may have a compulsion to cut myself, but I don't. Instead, I don't consciously do something, but I think that I might sit in such way that I know is going to give me a sore back later, or just ignore my body telling me to do something else. I might eat poorly [or] keep myself up so I get little sleep. At one point a friend pointed out that I was letting my cat scratch me a lot. . . . I pick my lip a lot, but I have always done that. . . . I'm not always as vigilant as I could be about getting the medical care that I need. . . . I don't think I get exactly the same thing out of [these passive ways] as I did when I was cutting myself or hitting myself, . . . but [I] think about those things as possibly alternative ways — that I haven't given up the desire to punish myself, I just have given up the overt behavior.

Sometimes I will [still] pick off scabs. A couple of summers ago I had a mosquito bite on my foot that was itchy and I scratched it so much that it formed a scab. One night as I was watching television, I picked it off and was surprised at how deep it was and how much blood was coming out. That was another time that I was feeling very numb — it wasn't an angry thing, it was a numbness thing. As I watched the blood I was like, "Wow! I am alive." I was fixated on it and decided I wanted to take photographs of it. So, I took photographs of my foot as it bled, and eventually the blood coagulated and stayed on my foot. So I just let myself be expressive, and I took pictures of my foot with all kinds of things: with this teddy bear that I had had when I was a child, with some jacks I used to play with when I was a kid, with some under-wear — anything I could think of that felt, at the moment, important to take a photograph of my foot with. Then . . . I took photographs of myself cleaning off my foot — [just] this disembodied hand and foot. I took photographs of myself with a new band-aid on it and then of my foot in a dress shoe so you could see the band-aid. I could have counted this as self-injury but didn't be-cause it wasn't the same. [Looking at the photographs didn't give me any kind of relief the way that picking or cutting would do.] I don't know why I took them; perhaps I thought I was being artistic. I definitely had it in my mind that I was [photographing my foot] with things that I associated with my childhood and the abuse.

Now, I feel less destructive and I can say that I haven't self-injured [for about four years], but I still have the compulsions to do it, very strongly sometimes. It's just that I am trying to be self-loving enough not to *do* it. The compulsion is more when I'm upset with myself and I have to hold myself back from putting my hand through the window. I have such rage, you know, usually at myself, I guess at times at other things. But I have so much energy [that gets] built up, built up, and I want so much to grab the knife, and I want to put my hand through the window, [and] I want to pound my fist through the wall — I want to *do* something physical. It is less now because — I don't know why actually, but before it would be the only thing that I could think about until I did it. And [now] I think about it, think about it, but even-tually it is okay and I don't think about it anymore. Or I try to do exercising, or punch the air, or swim vigorously, [or] walk on the treadmill [and] pump my arms — get the energy out some other way. That is harder and harder to do with my back. I'm having sciatica again, and I am very worried about it. So I haven't been able to do any vigorous exercise, anything aerobic where you really get your blood going and you're able to have that as a stress re-liever. I was not able to do that all my adult life [because of] back problems that began at around sixteen. I think that I channeled to [self-injury] some of [the feelings] that could have gotten channeled in other ways. People that have a disability like this have a harder time being able to use exercise.

It definitely feels like a compulsion, definitely feels like, "Do it, do it, do it, do it, do it." And I am like, "No, no, no, no — yes!" This is not the kind of thing that you can just call anybody up and say, "I'm thinking about hurting myself," because one of two things will happen: they will think that you are bananas and will not be able to deal with you, or think you are trying to com-mit suicide, which is a very different thing, and will call the police. So you have to be very picky. I do have a friend or two now who I can call and say,

"I really want to hurt myself. I am not going to do it — don't worry — just feeling like I want to and I need to talk to someone; I just need to tell you." But I haven't done that; I haven't talked to anybody about it. I just deal with it on my own. There are so many things wrong with me [and] there are only so many times you can call your friends.

I feel that having stopped makes it okay to tell other people. Now, I have friends who know. . . . I feel that if I was still doing it actively that it wouldn't be fair to be telling a lot of people because they can't do anything about it [unless they were] friends within the context of a support group. I refer to it as something that used to happen. . . . Not all of my friends know; I don't even know which of my friends does and doesn't. It is not something that I'm proud of but also it isn't something that I'm particularly ashamed of. I would certainly conceal it from prospective employers, but it isn't something that I feel I must hide at all costs from everyone.

I was talking to a friend this weekend. He is Buddhist and he was telling me about [a former] Buddhist practice of self-immolation. He says that in Buddhism they say that you should not practice any of this self-denial or self-injurious practices unless you already have a very high self-esteem or self-love. I thought that was very interesting. I don't know who on earth does have enough self-esteem that that would be okay, but I certainly speak from ignorance; I don't know very much about Buddhism.

It did remind me of something else. . . . I'm Jewish and I'm fairly observant, and Yom Kippur is a day where we are told to afflict ourselves. . . . The way that this injunction is carried out now is by fasting all day. You fast all day long and there are strictures: you don't wear leather, you don't wear jewelry, no perfume, and sexual relations are also prohibited. You can bathe to be clean but you don't bathe for pleasure. You are practicing self-denial, you are practicing self-affliction. And there is a point in the service when there's a long recitation of communal sins. . . . When you do this you ritually beat yourself on the breast: you take your right hand, make a fist, and hit yourself. Some people really whack themselves, and some people kind of do a tap. For a very long time I would *not* do that because I felt like I'm already hurting myself all the time. I still fasted and I did all the other things, but I didn't want to hit myself. But I also led the services, [and] up there in front of everybody I can't not do it. So I pretended to do it: I would put my hand up there and very lightly [do it]. And now that I have stopped self-injuring I do it again, I hit myself, I mean I beat myself, but I don't do it very hard.

This whole Day of Atonement, you know, beating up on yourself metaphysically: there are a lot of discussions in my . . . Jewish community about women doing these things. Women beat up on themselves and think that they are not okay all the time. So this idea of having one day where you do it to the hilt may not be such a hot idea. Women are always atoning; generally there is a trend for that. Being an abuse survivor, perhaps any kind of self-denial of my body is not so good. But now, before I start with the ritual beating of the breast, I rub the area that I am going to hit to sort of say, "I'm going to hit myself now, but I love myself, it's okay, I'm doing this ritual on purpose," and then I do it. When I'm done, I rub the area again, trying to be nurturing. So that's how I negotiate that particular thing now.

I don't *know* why [I was able to stop the cutting and hitting]. Wouldn't it be great if I did? If I could bottle that I'd give it away free. I don't have enough sense of a time when it stopped or the reason. It wasn't like one day I decided I'm not going to do this anymore. I suspect that it has to do with the fact that I have been in therapy forever, and that I have been working very hard on my self-esteem and on the way that I comport myself, just realizing that it's not a hot idea, that however much it may give me relief at the time, in the long run it's certainly doing me damage. It's a coping mechanism that I need to get rid of and replace with something which is healthier. It was the kind of thing where I was promising a therapist from this time to [next] time that I was not going to do it anymore. I used to do that occasionally with therapists. I guess I made a bargain with myself: "I am not going to do this anymore."

I'm not sure what I get out of [stopping]. . . . I guess I am supposed to get better mental health. I do it out of duty: I am not supposed to do this anymore, so I don't. But it isn't as if I do not wish to.

It's will power. [I don't mean it to] sound like "Oh, I can do this," or "I should have done it before," or "Other people should just be able to have will power." That's ridiculous. I couldn't have stopped before I stopped. . . . I was in a place where I needed that coping mechanism. I wasn't doing anything where I was going to die and I wasn't hurting anybody else. It wasn't good for me, but I did it and people do plenty of things that are bad for them. I'm not upset with myself, surprisingly. Since I tend to be so hard on myself about everything, it is amazing that I am not hard on myself about this.

[Now, when] I recognize I want to do it, I say, "Okay, I'm not going to do it," and turn my attention to other things if possible. I cook a lot; but for a lot of people cooking involves knives and sharp things. . . . But I cook in order to feel like a grownup and feel like I'm doing something productive, and it's distracting, and I like to cook, and I like to eat. . . . I cry a lot, and feel wretched, or I will make myself a cup of tea and watch mindless television, somehow figure out a way to numb out of it. Or I'll call my therapist. So, sometimes I will work the feeling, but often I feel like I don't have the sup port to do that, and so I will just numb it out and make it go away. Sometimes I'll call a friend, but not tell them that I want to hurt myself. I just get into a conversation with them and distract myself, having to constantly say [to myself], "You are not going to do this, okay? You are not going to do it; you are *not* going to do it."

One of my major coping mechanisms is to watch television [because] I also need mentally to distract myself. I eat some kind of comfort food and watch television, letting myself numb out, veg out so that I can get through it. It's the sort of one-hour thing: "I can go one more hour without hurting myself, I can go one more hour, I can go one *more* hour," and then fall asleep and get up in the morning. Sometimes I feel better and sometimes I feel worse, but usually by the morning I've slept it off and I get myself distracted with other things.

It's a time when the dissociation coping mechanism comes in handy because I let myself fan out and lift out and go away so I won't have these strong feelings to hurt myself: I'm not in my body wanting to do it. . . . Right now my life is so intolerable that it's much easier for me to be kind of, "This isn't really happening." . . . It's a way that I got through the abuse, it's a way that I get through difficult times now. I've got it in the back of my mind: "Through all of life's hardships—because there will be many more, no one can escape them—I will just dissociate; that's how I'll cope with them!" This is not good. I've got to figure out some other way to do it. However . . . dissociating works really well—divorce myself from my feelings—because even though it means I'm not feeling my feelings, it keeps me from hurting myself. What I really need to do is have feelings and be able to go to therapy at that time and deal with my feelings in a safe place. But I can't always do that, [and] . . . the dissociating gets me through. It is an interim measure. I continue to work on my self-esteem and my coping mechanisms so that dissociation won't be the coping mechanism anymore. Ultimately it's not so good.

But I should say that it's not as if I get a compulsion and then I go, "Okay, I know what to do: I'm going to do this and I'm going to do that and now everything's fine." It's so hard; I mean it's really, really difficult to do. My hands will actually *itch*; it's like "itchy fingers," you know, but it's a physical feeling like they're itching to do something and they're tingly. I feel like they're going to involuntarily reach out and do something. A lot of times I get a compulsion to punch the window in, knowing that it's going to cut me up, or hit the wall, or grab something and cut myself or scratch myself—*do* something. It's very, very strong. All the different ways I could hurt myself run through my mind and it's like, "Come on, let's go do it, let's go do it, let's go do it, let's go do it." And I really, really, really, really want to—and I just don't.

I remind myself, "Okay, you can't do this anymore; this is *bad*. If you do this, then you will backslide. Remember you're supposed to be loving yourself now. Let's go away to Borneo, fa-la-la-la-la. Let's watch television; yes, that's right, let's find something good on the television; and if there's nothing good on the television, we can watch this video that we like to watch when we're feeling yucky. And if you want to, you can have some chocolate or something that will make you feel like you are taking care of yourself"—although I really do try not to eat, but sometimes I do.

I think I'm more aware of [my hands itching] since I've stopped [injuring myself] than I ever was before because it wasn't that they were itching long: if I wanted to do it, I would just go do it. That was how I felt better; I wasn't trying to stop myself. So when I figured out that it wasn't such a great coping mechanism, then I felt the compulsion more because I felt it longer, because I wasn't doing the thing. And now, it goes on and on and on. . . .

Sometimes I do things that aren't so very good. . . . Sometimes I'm hungry: I have to eat or I feel I want to eat some kind of comfort food. I don't binge, but I feel that I'm really upset and I shouldn't be eating comfort food because I think it distorts things. I work very hard to not have food issues, and so I know that I'm doing a bad thing, and I worry that maybe it's another way of punishing myself, of injuring myself without actually doing it. I have a complex relationship to food and I used to binge-eat but I never purged. I used to do a lot of compulsive eating but never enough to make myself sick; it was never that bad, but it was always compulsive. I still have that sort of potential behavior lurking around, but I just don't do it anymore. . . . I'm trying to be aware of societal pressure to be a particular size, a particular shape, especially for women. I find it to be very oppressive, and I wish to get rid of that in myself.

[When I feel bad, I avoid] anything that has a double meaning for me, and sex definitely does, and food definitely does. Tea does not; I don't have any negative associations with tea, so if I want to have myself a nice nurturing cup of tea, fine. TV doesn't really, so if I want to watch television and zone out, that's what I do. But for me, sex and violence are all blurred up, and I don't want to blur them more. I try to avoid any sexual activity and that includes masturbation . . . because that just feeds it. I don't want to associate hurting myself with certain things that are supposed to be good and pleasurable. . . . I don't want to associate food with self-injury because I want food to be a nurturing thing for me.

I don't want to associate self-injury with alcohol because I don't want to develop alcoholism: I don't want to abuse myself *more*. Sometimes I do have a compulsion to have a drink and sometimes I do have a drink, but I've never been drunk in my life . . . I'd have just one drink. I really don't want to develop that. I know that my addictions can transfer, and I don't want them to. I have an addictive personality, you know: I was addicted to cutting myself, addicted to food, I don't want to become addicted to alcohol. . . . But I worry that I may transfer simply because the compulsion is still there, and the tendency, and the feelings that made me do these things before are still there. So, I'm working on all that: I'm a work in progress; aren't we all?

You know, you can make yourself not smoke, but you still want to smoke. It's harder to get rid of the compulsion to do it; I'm working on that now. I'm just starting to work with this new therapist who does a technique that's supposed to help people with phobias and addictions and negative associations between things. When I was talking with him about what I wanted to do, I thought, "What if I throw this in: Let's get rid of the compulsion to self-injure; that would be good." He does this thing called EMDR, which stands for eye-movement desensitization and reprocessing. He does a lot of mind/body stuff. Furthermore, he's a man, and I would never have thought in a million years that I would go to see a man for therapy. And here I am, seeing a man for therapy and I really liked him, but it brings up stuff that seeing a woman for therapy wouldn't. So I'm hoping to be able to use this therapy to, among other things, work on my compulsion, to figure out a way not to want to do it, although that may be impossible to completely avoid, because it's not a physical addiction the way smoking is or alcohol . . . there are emotional things that are situation-specific that make you want to do it. So, I'm never going to get rid of all those things; I'm never going to be able to avoid, for the whole rest of my life, feeling bad about myself or [other] triggers. . . .

If I [should] give in to the compulsion to hurt myself, I would feel that I had failed, that I was bad. For me it's very important in my ongoing quest for higher self-esteem *not* to do it. And I know that that's another reason why I don't do it anymore; why I'm vigilant about it even when it is very hard not to. You know, I have worked on myself very hard to get to the point where I felt that I could sustain a significant relationship and be a nurturing parent. Those are two very large goals in my life. I absolutely intend to become a parent, and since I feel that way, I absolutely intend to keep up with this not-hurting-myself stuff.

[My life has changed because I have stopped the most overt ways of injuring myself.] I'm no longer doing it: that's a change. I also feel that my friends were upset by this behavior, and I'm able to say, "I don't do this anymore; it's okay." I don't have to hide something; my friends don't have to worry that I'm doing it again. No one has to question, if I have a band-aid, did I do it myself or is this a cut from something else. So I feel that that makes me a more stable person. I'm not this crazy person doing this thing; I have got [it] under control. It's the same, I feel, as someone who is drinking too much and this can get in the way of relationships; it gets in the way of all kinds of things. . . . Everyone I know can trust me that I'm not going to do it anymore, and so no one has to worry about me; I'm stable, I'm not going to disappoint anyone, including myself. I also feel like it is something I feel good about, that I've accomplished, that I don't do it anymore. . . . I don't have to worry that I'm going to do this behavior once I have children, that they're going to witness this. I don't have to worry that I shouldn't have them because I have this thing. I *did* that; I have gotten over that.

But I would reword [your] question [about whether my life has changed since I stopped injuring myself]. The way I would reword it is: Can I envision a time when I don't have the compulsion? Would my life be different if I didn't *want* to do this? And [the answer is that] it would be much better. I mean, it would be just great if I could get rid of the compulsion to do it because it takes a *lot* of energy not to do it: I'm exhausted by it. I really *hate* it when I feel compelled to do it because I want to do it and I know that I'm not going to, and so I sit around going, "God, this is terrible, I hate this." I'm denying myself the way I know I will feel better in the short term. I *know* that if I do it that the feeling will be better, but I also know that in the long term it's not a good idea. And it's not that it's constant, but when it does happen, I'm like, "Oh great, now I'm going to have to put all this energy into not doing it," because it takes tremendous willpower not to do it. And I'm very proud of myself when I don't, but I'm dismayed every time I feel like I want to: "Ugh, I can't believe this. Now I can't eat anything, now I have to expend all this energy and I'd really rather do something else." And also the fact that I want to hurt myself means that I still harbor all this self-hatred and shame and [other] reasons that I would want to hurt myself. So it would be lovely to get rid of that, too, or at least to have it be less of an ugly monster.

And I do worry about the future . . . because we all suffer in life; we all go through terrible tragedies; we all face things that seem unbearable. This is a coping mechanism for me. Will I return to it? I certainly hope not. But I have not experienced the greatest tragedies of life. I've certainly experienced some of the really nasty ones, but who knows what's out there waiting for me, for any of us. And as long as I know that this coping mechanism does make me feel better in the short term, it's technically on the table, and I'd like for it not to be on the table. I'd like to know for certain I'm not going to do that anymore. And the only way I can know for certain now is just to keep promising myself and those around me that I won't. But people return to their addictive behaviors all the time when they're under enormous amounts of stress and pain. And I hope that I won't be one of those people, but I'm no greater or lesser than anyone else and I'm certainly susceptible to those tendencies. So I can only say that I hope I won't.

7 Help for Women Who Self-Injure and Their Therapists

EVEN WHEN self-injury has been a coping mechanism for many years, a woman does not have to think that she will always need it. Recovery is possible and can occur in gradations, such as learning to feel less overwhelmed by self-injury, lessening the frequency or degree of self-injury, stopping one type of self-injury but continuing others, stopping altogether even though the urge recurs, and stopping altogether with no recurrent urge to self-injure. Many women have experienced such changes, giving hope to others. Alleviating and then stopping self-injury takes time, often many years. When a woman is able to stop, the reasons are often difficult to pinpoint. It seems crucial for a woman to be prepared to work hard and to utilize self-help and competent professional guidance. My informants' experiences may help women looking for ways to stop and may also be of interest to therapists who want to help self-injuring women.

Self-Help Methods

Self-help methods for delaying or stopping self-injury are familiar topics to my informants. All have used self-help, and the methods they have used as well as those used by other self-injuring women [1] illustrate that self-help methods can be as diverse as the women who self-injure. One woman's help may be another woman's horror: even a simple relaxation exercise can be soothing for some and intolerable for others. A woman may not know which methods are best for her until she tries them. Many techniques are applicable to several types of self-injury—such as cutting, hitting, burning, or picking—and some are specific to a single type. Among the suggestions listed in this chapter, women can choose any they think might help them and add ideas of their own. Additional ideas may be gleaned from the resources listed in the back of this book.

Be aware that you may find some or all of the following suggestions difficult to carry out. With each suggestion, give yourself permission not to be able to do it, or to do only increments of it. Also, give yourself credit for each time you are able to refrain from injuring yourself, or for having a longer than usual period free of self-injury:

1. Remember that many other people injure themselves. You are not alone and not a "freak."

2. Try to set aside guilt and shame about injuring yourself. Instead, allow yourself to admit that self-injury indicates a problem.

3. Be kind to yourself in as many ways as possible, including treating your body well. Keep a consistent 24-hour rhythm of activity, sleep, and healthy eating. You may find that having a professional massage, or having a friend or partner give you a back rub or massage, can help relieve anxiety. Rosa rubs vitamin E oil into her skin after a bath. She finds that the oil helps her scars to fade and that caring for her skin is the opposite of injuring herself. She also gives herself a manicure, an act of self-caring that helps her refrain from biting and tearing at her cuticles. Smoothing the callouses on the bottom of her feet with a pumice stone helps keep her from tearing at and cutting her soles, her favorite place for cutting. The smoothness of her soles makes it less tempting for her to cut and tear them, and the working action of the pumice stone is similar to and a substitute for tearing and cutting.

4. Be gentle with yourself mentally as well as physically. Forgive your own blunders, errors, faults, and compulsions. Try to see them as experiences to learn from and challenges to surmount.

5. Try making positive statements about yourself. Start off by writing five things that you find good about yourself, then find ten new ones. Elizabeth found that she had to look hard for good attributes but that it was worth the effort: "It kind of tunes you in to, 'Oh, there are some good things about me.'" She still has her list of affirmations and can look at them repeatedly to remind herself of her good qualities.

6. Do healthful things that are pleasurable and help keep negative thoughts at bay. Karen reads things that she loves and that distract and move her in positive ways. Sometimes she dances by herself to music or has fun with her daughter. When she knows that her husband and children will be away, she tries to call someone or have someone around the house so that negative thoughts will not take over. Like many women living with the aftermath of childhood abuse, Karen finds loneliness and boredom intolerable because they encourage rumination. For some women, seeing a movie, watching TV, petting and playing with an animal, taking a hot bath or shower, having a nap, drawing, painting, playing a musical instrument, or just listening to music may soothe away or distract from the need to self-injure.

7. Keep a store of comforting images or objects to draw upon. Have self-

soothing objects on hand, such as very small stuffed animals for a purse or pocket. Esther keeps little rocks and figurines — her "comfort items" — at her workplace. Sometimes she can reach for them instead of injuring herself. Erica carries pictures of her cat in her head: he is her "touchstone," and his image makes her feel good.

8. Nature can be soothing. Peggy finds that seeing things come alive in the spring eases her life's strains. Esther has the good fortune of living near a wooded reservoir where she can walk and observe the ducks and geese. She also goes to the ocean now and then where she relaxes by walking along the beach, enjoying the smell and sound of the ocean and the reminder that "there's something bigger." Throwing stones into water can sometimes bring release. Erica was once on vacation at a coastal area full of wildflowers, birds, and beautiful woods. While there, a child came to visit her, and Erica became caught up in the child's world, finding peace of mind.

9. Relaxation exercises, such as deep breathing and visualizing peaceful scenes, may help reduce anxiety. Be aware, however, that for some abused women such exercises increase anxiety because distressing images, thoughts, or feelings intrude, or because a woman begins to experience her body in disturbing ways.

10. Improve the quality of your life in as many ways as possible. For Erica, one important factor in possible recovery is building a life that she wants: a job she enjoys, a pleasurable social life, confidants with whom she can talk about trying to stop. All these components help her feel less alienated.

11. Find a place in your environment or imagination where you feel safe from harm. Erica had a remarkable feeling of liberation when her parents sold the house in which they had lived since her birth. Now, she will never again have to go to that place still associated in her mind with danger. Erica also worked hard to establish "safe places" in her mind. Sometimes she uses images of leaving, escaping, or disappearing to piece together comforting fantasies. These include fantasies of getting into a car and driving, hiding in the attic, and being rescued by neighbors from abusive parents. She also imagines herself cuddling with her partner, or talking with her therapist — not about cutting, just talking in general.

12. When you feel the urge to injure yourself, try calling a friend, a therapist, or a sponsor. The important aspect of the call is not necessarily to talk about your urge or about why you want to self-injure, but to delay self-injury and distract yourself until you can "get over the hump." Some women call friends who know nothing about the self-injury and simply chat or invent a reason for having called. If you call your therapist, even talking to her or his answering machine can be a useful delay tactic. If you plan to repeatedly call

someone who knows about your self-injury, you may want to discuss with her/ him during a relaxed moment things that would be useful for the person to ask or say in acute situations. You may also prefer being with someone rather than talking on the phone, or prefer corresponding with a trusted friend by letter, email, or the internet.

13. Ask your therapist, sponsor, or other confidant to make a tape reminding you of her or his presence and your relationship to each other. Listening to the tape may help if you find it hard to believe in an absent person's existence in your life. A tape of stories or poems in this person's voice may serve as a soothing reminder.

14. Movement can be useful in many ways. Going for a walk, running, dancing, swimming, punching the air or a punching bag, working out, cleaning the house, or pacing the room can release energy, relieve boredom, and perhaps release internal, soothing chemicals called endorphins, all of which can alleviate the urge to self-injure. Meredith sometimes plays catch with a friend and throws the ball hard. She finds that this "gets those feelings out" and tires her. When walking, running, or swimming, you might try imagining that you are leaving everything negative behind you, or that the wind is blowing them out of your mind and body. (Remember that movement by driving a car is not always a safe way to release energy, and driving may be better used as transportation to the gym or pool, not as a release in itself.)

15. If the sight of knives or razors triggers an urge to cut yourself, try banning them or putting them where they are hard to reach and buying all your food precut.

16. Keeping your hands busy by writing in a journal, painting, or sculpting can be useful distractions and may also help you understand and express the feelings that lead to self-injury. Other activities that divert your hands are knitting, crocheting, doodling, ripping paper, or playing with beads. Often, your thoughts as well as your hands will need to be distracted. You may find, however, that digging into something with a pen and scribbling hard can keep you from digging into your skin. You may also avoid cutting yourself by throwing clay against something, slamming doors, beating on a drum, hammering nails into a board, or "injuring" a stuffed animal, especially when the overriding emotion is rage. When trying these and other alternatives it can be useful to allow no razors in your house, and to keep a barrier of thick clothing on parts of your body that you habitually injure.

17. Take a course in assertiveness and/or anger management to help you learn to stand up for yourself and both control and safely express explosive anger. You can also practice on your own, perhaps with the aid of self-help books. Barbara sometimes makes an "angry" sculpture or finds that the act of

sculpting itself alleviates her anger. She also asks close friends to loosely roll her in a futon and hold her so that she can scream and thrash without hurting herself or others. Caroline is "learning how to be adult" by telling herself, "It'll move in a minute" when stuck in traffic, or telling a friend that she is angry with her. These are better responses than banging on the steering wheel in self-injurious frustration, or exploding at a friend, then injuring herself in self-blame for having hurt someone else. During less acute anger, simply express-ing feelings verbally may help deflect an escalation leading to self-injury.

18. Holding an ice cube or cold pack against your skin may help deflect the urge to cut because the burning sensation of ice is similar to the sensation of the wound after cutting. If your urge is to cut or pick, you can also try holding an ice cube in your hand or plunging your arm into a bucket of icy water and leaving it for a minute. General intense sensations may be useful, such as biting into hot peppers or rubbing VapoRub under your nose. Other possible cutting substitutes are using a red, water-based, nontoxic marker on your skin, or putting a rubber band on your wrist and pulling on it constantly for two minutes.

19. If you need to feel physical pain, you can try standing on your toes until pain comes. (Some women are uneasy with this suggestion because it is a form of self-injury, though socially acceptable and less obvious.)

20. Carrying around a picture of yourself as a baby may help, after remind-ing yourself how you would protect and care for a baby girl entrusted to you.

21. Some women find that they can talk themselves out of self-injury, at least for a while, especially if they can catch themselves before the urge to injure becomes overpowering: "I'm not going to do anything for half an hour"; "I'll not get myself ready by taking off my clothes, then I won't want to do it because it will ruin my clothes"; "When I get home I can cut"; "I won't do it because I don't have any band-aids" or "because I don't want my children to see me with cuts" or "because I don't want to disappoint my therapist." You might try identifying what you feel, then telling yourself things you need to hear: "It's okay, you're safe," or "My error isn't the end of the world. I'll try to do better next time." Now, when Peggy thinks about banging her head she says to herself, "No, I like myself too much to hurt myself." Meredith tells herself, "Okay, these are just feelings; you don't have to act on them." Other possibili-ties include "I am lovable," "I am not alone," and "I can recover." Even count-ing to ten may defuse an impending explosion. When talking to yourself seems inadequate, screaming or crying may bring relief. Women who believe in a higher power sometimes pray for help.

22. Members of support groups can sometimes help each other abstain from self-injury. If a group such as Alcoholics Anonymous, Overeaters Anony-

mous, Narcotics Anonymous, or Survivors of Incest Anonymous applies to you and you feel comfortable with their programs, members may help you refrain from self-injury and bring you together with other self-injuring women. Some reminders from such 12-step programs — such as "One day (or one hour) at a time" — can also be useful. To find a support group specifically for self-injury, contact a women's center, hospital, or mental health facility near you. They may know of one, if not for self-injury specifically, then one for women who have experienced incest or other childhood abuses (if they apply to you). They may also be willing to post a flier to help you start a self-injury support group if none exists in your area, and they should be able to help you locate 12-step and other support groups that deal with various problems. You can also make connections on the internet or join an already existing internet group. (See the resources at the end of this book for more information on using the internet.)

23. If you have internet access, you can email your postal mailing address to llama@palace.net and receive tokens for thirty, sixty, and so on days free of self-injury. The tokens can help encourage your efforts to stop, and remind you that you are not alone. If you stop self-injuring for a while and then start again, avoid focusing on the slip ("I had sixty days and now I'm at day one again") and instead use the tokens to acknowledge your achievement: "I've only injured once in two months. I really *can* stop."[2]

24. Some women find that having a written or verbal agreement with their therapists not to cut themselves helps them refrain from cutting, although they may injure themselves in other ways instead. This is a delay tactic that is either very helpful or very harmful, and some women advise against it, as discussed later in this chapter.

25. Finally, a last resort to keep yourself from self-injury would be to go into a hospital if past experiences with hospitalizations have been positive. Sometimes Jane, who has been treated well during hospitalizations, uses this tactic to keep herself from cutting. She knows the staff members and hospital routine and does not fear them, whereas she does sometimes fear her own cutting.

You may want to make a self-help package containing a list of alternatives to self-injury, soothing objects, telephone numbers of resource people, comforting audiotapes, photos that remind you of the present or of special people, and other useful items, and keep the package where you can easily find it in times of stress.

Barbara is an example of a woman in the process of trying to overcome self-injury who has used some of the methods mentioned above to help her get through her emotions — even rage — without injuring herself. Barbara once thought that if she did not cut herself, she would die. She felt as though her feelings could kill her unless she fled into dissociation, released them through cutting, or both. She thinks that "early training" in dissociation evolved into taking drugs and cutting herself as ways of surviving emotions that felt lethal. After sixteen years of self-help and professional help, and of attending meetings with Alcoholics Anonymous, Narcotics Anonymous, and Survivors of Incest Anonymous groups, Barbara now allows herself to feel her emotions, realizing that she can endure them and survive. Each time she lives through the intensity of her emotions, she feels stronger.

Barbara acknowledges that she sometimes relapses, but when that happens she tells herself, "I had a slip and have to try again to abstain from it." She tries to look at the progress she has made, find out where she went wrong, and plan to do something different next time. She now has a commitment to stay in the present rather than escape. It is her life, she says, and "life isn't always pretty but it doesn't mean you can check out; it means you hang in there and it will pass." She has learned that the feelings she thought she had to change will change on their own if only she can bear them until they do. If she intervenes, she misses an opportunity to empower herself by living through the experience. "But sometimes I don't care," she says, acknowledging that her emotions still occasionally overpower her.

As part of her recovery, Barbara feels accountable for overcoming self-injury. This is why she reminds herself of every time she gets through difficulties without picking up a razor blade. Nowadays, Barbara considers self-cutting episodes "slips" and focuses on the way that days free from self-injury accumulate into weeks. Each stressful situation she goes through without cutting strengthens her for future stresses:

. . . .

When I'm dying to pick up a razor blade — like it is so far in my body that I can taste it I want to do it so bad — if I sit through one of those times without doing it, then I get the strength to say, "Remember you got through that time without it."

. . . .

In the past while cutting herself, Barbara thought only of the relief it was bringing and was glad to be able to feel better: "There was a rightness about it. I felt like, 'Oh good, now I am getting to be real about what is going on. Now, I get to mark physically what's going on emotionally.'" When she felt split, cutting would pull the parts of her together. Afterward, she felt a peacefulness, a resolution. Lately, when she cuts herself she thinks, "I wish I didn't have to be doing this." Although the cutting still often gives her what she needs, afterward she feels a regretful disappointment and asks herself, "Why didn't I try to call someone?" Cutting also hurts now whereas it usually did not before, perhaps suggesting that she dissociates less severely, an encouraging sign.

Barbara can envision living without self-injury, but only day by day; it is still too frightening to think of a lifetime without it. She tries not to think too far ahead, instead making a commitment each morning not to injure herself that day. Having overcome alcohol and other drug addictions "a day at a time," she is trying the same technique with self-injury—a technique that can be useful for women familiar with addictions. On some days, the commitment to stop is difficult because self-injury is constantly on her mind. If she feels rushed and stressed, she wants to self-injure to "take the edge off," just as alcohol used to do.

Each time Barbara refrains from self-injury, her life changes: she has to confront stressful situations and her feelings rather than escape through self-injury. She asks herself, "What am I really *feeling* right now? If I'm cutting, what am I trying to say?" Barbara is getting to know her own feelings and sometimes engages in conflict and confronts other people. She thinks that these changes will eventually lead to a more productive life.

Talk Therapy

Along with self-help, Barbara, like many women, has had extensive professional help to try to better understand why she injures herself and to decrease and eventually stop self-injury. Talk therapy, individually or in groups, is usually part of such professional help. Yet, few studies of talk therapy specifically address self-injury and those that do usually have inconclusive results, not surprising given self-injury's great complexity. Studies of such therapies are short relative to the years recovery can require and are restricted to, for example, groups of women diagnosed as having borderline personality disorder or those who have been in psychiatric hospitals or residential treatment centers. Therefore, in making therapy choices it helps to know what types of therapies are available, to read about other self-injuring women's experiences with therapy, and to learn what qualities others have found important in a therapist.

Some form of talk therapy, sometimes two types or more, seems to be the crux of professional help for experiences and behaviors that have been unspoken and unspeakable for years. This is true even when the initial therapy sessions—or even the first few years of therapy—go by without mention of self-injury or prior abuse. In fact, many (perhaps most) self-injuring women do not initially seek therapy for self-injury but for depression, anxiety, body pains, or other problems. Eventually, however, self-injury may emerge as a topic of discussion, and incidents of self-injury can slowly decrease after an abused woman's past has been gently explored and understood, and as her life options increase,[3] leaving her with a sense of empowerment over her past and present.

Talk therapy can take place in individual, group, or family settings, and therapists can have different perspectives — such as psychodynamic, developmental, cognitive-behavioral, feminist, solution-oriented, and interpersonal, among others — that influence how they work. Most good therapists are eclectic to some degree even if they lean toward a particular model: they have to be flexible to meet their clients' needs.

All my informants were using individual talk-therapy at the time of the interviews. All women found some of it beneficial, though their enthusiasm varied. A few went through long periods of useless or harmful therapy sessions before finding knowledgeable, skilled, compatible therapists.

Therapy can be helpful even though the client is not sure why. Sometimes, though, women were able to name specific aspects of therapy that they found helpful. First of all, talking with a therapist is often a self-injuring woman's first break in silence and isolation: this alone is an important step toward recovery. Also, repeated sessions with an empathetic, skilled therapist can build self-esteem because a woman sees that her therapist stays with her through emotionally turbulent times. As Barbara says:

. . . .

After a lot of therapy, I realized that I deserve to have intimate relationships and they weren't necessarily going to turn out like the ones in my past. . . . I had seven years with one therapist, two with another, and seven years with another. . . . We went through thick and thin together and they stuck by me. . . . Anyone can stand you for one hour a week for a year, but when it's two hours a week times seven years, it's like wow! — and the phone calls in between. I guess I'm not unlovable if this person hung in there with me.

. . . .

Such a relationship can help a woman learn to trust another person's goodwill and benignity, especially important for women previously abused by people they trusted and upon whom their welfare depended. Talking about past abuses can help a woman validate and work through those experiences, integrating them as much as possible into her life's history and acknowledging their continuing effects, such as self-hatred, dissociation, and self-injury. Discussing current problems can help put them into perspective and differentiate them from past experiences.

All these aspects of therapy can potentially help a women build a satisfying life for herself with goals, obligations, and relationships. Self-injury may be easier to overcome as a result. In the framework of strengthening trust and self-esteem, a therapist can help a woman look at the thoughts and emotions that precede self-injury and try to understand them. Some women have sessions with a cognitive-behavioral therapist who specializes in helping to identify thoughts that can lead to self-injury and to substitute them with thoughts that may reduce or check painful feelings and the need to self-injure. Therapist and client together can try to discover alternate ways of releasing the energy previously released through self-injury and ultimately, perhaps, substitute constructive activities such as vigorous movement, painting, playing an instrument, talking, or writing.

A woman may, however, find only some of her individual talk therapy useful, or find that she has to educate her therapist about self-injury before the therapy becomes helpful. One woman I talked to found that therapy seemed to help for a while but that in time, self-injury worsened. Self-injury can increase during therapy because painful feelings may come up or new memories emerge. Client and therapist may accept the increased self-injury as a necessary and temporary sign that core issues are being approached or addressed, and feel that the discussions of past events are safe, essential, and beneficial in the long term.

Group talk therapy has the same potential pitfalls and benefits as individual talk therapy with the additional requirement that trust and rapport must be built among group members. Even if it serves no other purpose, a talk therapy group (or a self-help group) can relieve each participant's feelings of being the only woman in the world who does these "strange things," an important step in itself. In a successful group, a woman can appreciate the facilitator's knowledge and skill and enjoy the solace of talking with other women who have the same or similar experiences and who can say, "I know what you mean" or "That's exactly how I feel."

One type of talk therapy, called dialectical behavior therapy, or DBT, specifically addresses self-injury. DBT is a subtype of cognitive behavior therapy conceived by Marsha Linehan for people diagnosed as having borderline personality disorder, a diagnostic label often attached to women who self-injure. As part of DBT, women work in groups toward learning specific skills to try to improve their relationships with others, regulate their emotions, tolerate distress, and manage their lives. Group members learn about coping skills, and discuss and practice those skills, consulting with a therapist on integrating the skills into daily life. One common DBT topic addresses using other coping solutions to replace self-injury, drug abuse, and other releases, including attempted suicide. In some treatment settings, all DBT takes place in groups and consultations by phone, while in other settings, individual therapy is part of DBT.

None of my informants had tried DBT, although Erica went to one group therapy session using DBT techniques and found that its approach was not for her. Other women, however, have reported that DBT gives them a welcome sense of autonomy while they are trying to decrease self-injury.[4] Therapists and clients not specifically using DBT often draw on skill development, a component of DBT, in working with intense and complex feelings. DBT techniques can be useful even when a woman deplores and rejects the diagnosis of borderline personality disorder. The University of Washington Department of Psychology, listed in the resources at the end of this book, may be able to help you find a DBT-trained therapist in your area.

Prescribed Psychotropic Drugs

Mind-altering (psychotropic) prescription drugs may help with depression and anxiety and may be tried along with some type of talk therapy. Only one of my informants, Barbara, mentioned such drugs as helping her resist self-injury. Many women who self-injure take a variety of prescribed mind-altering drugs in the hope that the drugs will subdue intense emotions, alleviate depression, or check impulsive reactions to stress. For some people, such a drug seems to help reduce the frequency of or temporarily halt self-injury. No studies of psychotropic drugs used in self-injury therapy are conclusive, and only anecdotes suggest that any certain drug or combination can help some women stop self-injury altogether.[5] Some researchers consider fluoxetine (Prozac), sertraline (Zoloft), paroxetine (Paxil), and fluvoxamine (Luvox), or other SSRIs (selective serotonin re-uptake inhibitors) most promising.[6] They can lose their effectiveness over time, however, and all can have unwanted effects such as headache, nausea, and anxiety.

Expressive Therapies

The purpose of expressive therapy is to express unspoken and perhaps unconscious thoughts and feelings in order to foster self-awareness and reconcile emotional conflicts. Drawing, painting, and sculpting are examples that employ shapes, forms, and colors that, along with the artist's own comments about the artwork, can be revealing statements about her past or present. A person can become acquainted with self-expression through music and dance, experiencing movement as a release or perhaps learning to play an instrument that becomes a lifelong source of pleasure and self-expression. Listening to certain musical tones can be soothing or releasing, and a skilled music therapist knows and uses the emotional qualities of tones and instruments. Acting, using the spoken word or mime, can allow personal expression disguised as playing a role. Keeping a personal journal (journaling) of thoughts, feelings, ideas, dreams, memories, events, or anything one wishes encourages self-expression through words and can help a person understand her actions and emotions and remember her feelings and dreams. Copying parts of the journal for a therapist can be a way of revealing things too painful to speak of face to face. Free-writing, line poems, word-clustering, and other associative word games can, with the help of a skilled therapist, bring useful discoveries of meanings and help lead to a habit of expression through words.[7]

Massage Therapy and Other Forms of Body Work

Massage therapy is simply massage: the manipulation of soft tissues using the hands or sometimes the forearms or elbows to apply fixed or moveable pressure and to hold or move the client's body. Other than relaxation, a goal of massage is to help release emotions or memories lodged partly in the body, especially among women who experienced childhood physical or sexual abuse. However, for exactly these reasons massage can be difficult or impossible to tolerate or make a woman feel worse afterward.

Women who have experienced childhood abuse can find other forms of body work helpful, some of which do not involve touch. These include Feldenkrais movements, Alexander techniques, acupressure/acupuncture, the Rubenfeld Synergy Method, Neuro-Emotional Treatment (done by chiropractors), and others. When considering any type of body work, make sure that the therapist is licensed, experienced in working with abused women, and knows how to react if the work releases memories. In any case, if you feel uncomfortable, remember that you are free to end the session and/or not to return.

Brief Trauma Therapies

Eye Movement Desensitization and Reprocessing (EMDR)

The client visualizes a traumatic scene and identifies a negative belief—for example, "It was my fault"—associated with it. Her eyes follow the therapist's finger as it makes rapid diagonal or horizontal sweeps, then shuts off the traumatic scene. Some therapists leave out the eye movements[8] but use alternating sounds or hand taps. EMDR often helps people overcome overwhelming anxiety or other negative emotions[9] while remembering traumatic events, and reduces their anxiety, depression, intrusive thoughts, and avoidance of trauma-associated situations.[10] One study showed that EMDR was equally effective with sexual, physical, and emotional abuse and that its effectiveness still held three months after the treatment.[11] No studies to date mention self-injury, but some therapists have found that EMDR helps their clients stop injuring themselves.[12]

A variety of other brief therapies, such as the three mentioned below,[13] seem to help many trauma victims decrease the response to thoughts and memories of a trauma. No one yet knows exactly why these therapies sometimes help or whether they can be useful in reducing or stopping self-injury.

Visual-Kinesthetic Dissociation

The client imagines watching her- or himself looking at a movie of a traumatic scene from beginning to end, then from the end to the beginning. The therapist then asks the client what new knowledge s/he has about the event and requests that s/he take that knowledge to the younger self who experienced the trauma.

Trauma Incident Reduction

The facilitator asks questions about the trauma and gives directions for picturing, with closed eyes, a traumatic scene, then describing the scene to the facilitator, and telling the facilitator how the incident seems now. The session consists of numerous repetitions of this process, dealing with only one traumatic episode at a time.

Thought Field Therapy

While thinking about a traumatic event, clients tap specific points on their bodies in a step-by-step sequence sometimes accompanied by eye movements, humming a tune, and counting. This therapy is based on the theory that energy flows along meridians and can be balanced and released by contact on acupressure points.

The types of therapies you try should be compatible to you, but their compatibility can depend largely on the therapist. Your choice of therapist, especially for talk therapies, could have the greatest consequence to your progress. Some therapists' beliefs, attitudes, and practices can cause a woman to feel worse about herself. Because not all caregivers are knowledgeable about self-injury, some react to it perplexedly, angrily, and punitively. Self-injuring women have been yelled at because of an injury; humiliated by having a caregiver ask others, in the woman's presence, how she can do this to herself; and threatened with hospitalization or desertion if she self-injures. These reactions can reinforce a woman's belief that she is "bad" and can confirm childhood traumatic experiences of having caregivers confine her against her will, shame her, or abandon her.

The diagnostic labels that caregivers employ for psychological problems can be validating, such as posttraumatic stress disorder, which blames an event rather than its victim; neutral, such as depression, which vaguely connotes a state of mind; or pejorative, such as borderline personality disorder, which blames the client by implying that her "personality" is at fault. Borderline personality disorder's negative connotations among professionals are so entrenched and widespread that self-injuring women who are therapists (and many who are not) are uneasy with or angry at the label and at the assumptions that often accompany it. In the official American categories of mental distress, borderline personality disorder (BPD) is the only diagnosis that specifies self-mutilating behavior as a criterion. It is one of nine criteria, of which five or more are necessary for the BPD diagnosis.[14] Some therapists may feel pressure to use the diagnosis of BPD in order to have their work taken seriously among professional peers. Yet, several of my informants objected to being viewed through the lens of BPD, a diagnosis they find misleading, demeaning, and often harmful to their chances of optimal care.

Many self-injuring women seeking help are asked to make safety contracts — written or verbal agreements between therapist and client — to refrain from self-injury. The term "safety contract" reflects two misconceptions: a woman can stop injuring herself at will, and self-cutting is a suicide attempt. The result of such a contract can be more frequent or more severe self-injury. The client often cannot refrain from self-injury, feels ashamed that she has "failed" to abide by the contract, and injures herself even more because the feeling of shame — already familiar to her — is intolerable. For women who frequently and almost unconsciously hit or pick at themselves, such contracts may impose an increase in pressure by taking away the minute-by-minute safety valve of self-injury. In psychiatric hospitals, breaking such contracts can lead to being involuntarily put in restraints, often a humiliating and enraging experience that can feel like a reenactment of childhood abuse. Being asked to sign a safety contract can feel like the equivalent of telling an alcoholic, "I will help you stop drinking, but first you must promise to stop drinking." Although some women have reached a point at which such contracts provide welcome and needed boundaries for their behavior, and help them keep their resolve not to injure themselves, others find that safety contracts make them feel as though they were "bad" and out of control, some of the feelings therapy is meant to alleviate.

Safety contracts are often created out of a fear of suicide. It is essential that caregivers understand that self-cutting is a lifesaving act, not attempted suicide. It is also essential that self-injuring women understand why therapists cannot easily lay the suicide question to rest. A recurring wish to die is part of the lives of many self-injuring women. The majority of women I talked with have had such thoughts, and several have attempted suicide at least once. In fact, the first episode of what becomes chronic cutting may occur shortly after an attempt to die, as though a woman had found an alternative to suicide. Some women say that during a suicide attempt through wrist-cutting, they realized that the cutting made them feel so much better they no longer wanted to die. Self-cutting, even of the wrist, then becomes a way to refrain from suicide. Unfortunately, the link between cutting and a prior suicide attempt can lead families and caregivers to interpret self-cutting as another attempt to die rather than as a way to stay alive. Some women say that not cutting for a long time makes them feel like attempting suicide. As Esther says, "I think it's a whole lot better to cut myself than to *kill* myself. And sometimes that's what it feels like: either I'm going to cut myself or I would rather not live."

A similar misunderstanding is the view that self-injury is a suicide attempt calculated to fail in order to gain a response from others. This misconception may partly explain why some therapists consider most self-injury "manipulative," a pejorative term found in professional journal articles. Also, caregivers and family members may feel that a woman who self-injures is doing it *to them* rather than *for herself* because they cannot understand why she would find such actions necessary.

Elizabeth, Jane, and Barbara sometimes want to die but not by the blade, and their actual suicide attempts have always been through medication overdoses. Nonetheless, all three suspect that they could be at risk of inadvertently killing themselves by cutting too deeply. Aware of this risk, Barbara switched to burning herself for a while. At times, when she has wanted to cut to the bone, she has driven to the hospital and cut herself in the parking lot so that she could get help before bleeding to death. Once she even cut in the hospital restroom, fearing that she might otherwise collapse from blood loss and die before she could get help. Such careful planning shows that Barbara wants to stay alive in spite of an act that so closely resembles an attempt to die.

A woman who self-injures may have alter identities, and these identities may do the cutting. Can they be trusted not to kill? One of Jane's alter identities is frequently either suicidal or homicidal. Jane thinks that this identity does not understand that if she kills Jane, she kills herself, and vice versa. An alter identity nearly severed a vein, suggesting that for Jane, inadvertent suicide by cutting is a genuine danger. Although Jane usually cuts strictly for release, she once planned to cut and lose blood daily while eating little, allowing herself time to get things in order before dying. Mary also has a suicidal alter identity, a child who cuts deeply, as opposed to other alter identities who are satisfied with a scratch and just a bit of blood. Therefore, Mary and her therapist are seemingly caught in a dilemma: dealing with an action that helps keep Mary alive, while worrying about the possibility of a fatal cut.

Possibly because of suicidal alter identities, some women who self-injure periodically play with the possibility of death:

. . . .

Elizabeth: I know that if I was cutting on the underside of my arm, that I would be dead by now. I know, because I go so deep that if I did it on this side I would have hit an artery. But sometimes then, that kind of tempts me to try it out: "Well, it wouldn't really be suicide, it would just be accidental"; I try to convince myself of that. But I always do it on the upper part of my forearm, and my upper arm, and my thighs. I always go here, I don't know why; it's always right below the elbow on my forearm.

. . . .

Elizabeth's teasing thoughts reveal the idea of suicide even though she has never cut the underside of her arm, and her actual suicide attempts have not been by cutting. Barbara uses the term "Russian roulette" to describe her gambles with death. She equates her reckless driving with cutting to the point that she could bleed to death. Even when she does not actually feel suicidal, there are times when she feels a need to play with death. At these moments, she feels that it would be alright if her car went off the cliff or if she bled to death. The risk itself seems necessary to release her from a dissociated state, leading to actions in which returning to life is accomplished by playing with death.

These experiences suggest that some women who self-injure could die accidentally by cutting, a source of anxiety for therapists, family members, and friends. Yet, no one can or should try to prevent a self-injuring woman from continuing to cut herself unless she feels ready and willing to make the effort. Sarah O. speaks for many self-cutting women when she says:

. . . .

Every therapist that I ever went to would make me contract for safety, you know, suicide-prevention stuff. And it's not suicidal, it's very different. For me it wasn't necessarily that I wanted to die, it was more problems with hating myself. I spent a lot of time in therapy paying people money to worry that I was going to kill myself, and that was not the case. What I really needed was [for them] to leave me alone and start dealing with some of the issues that were behind the cutting. It wasn't something that needed to be stopped immediately, [and] it wasn't going to stop by worrying about my immediate safety; it was only going to stop by working through some stuff. . . . Nothing was going to get better until I dealt with the issues, and sitting in therapy and talking about suicidality wasn't going to help me stop.

. . . .

Yet, because of the ethical dilemma posed to therapists for whom suicide is a feared occurrence, some therapists and clients find that contracts to call the therapist before cutting are a reasonable compromise.

In addition to knowing about harmful and controversial topics, it can be useful to know what other self-injuring women like and want in a therapist. A therapist's behaviors and attitudes can be more important than prescribing certain medications or using a particular therapeutic technique. My informants and other advocates find the following therapist attributes most productive:

- *Focusing on the individual thoughts, feelings, and events that lead a person to self-injure, not on self-injury itself.*

  Esther: React with concern, but not with concern about the injuries but what's *behind* them. I once cut up my hands a little, and I thought to myself at the time, "Why are you cutting your hands? People are going to see that." And I tried to tell myself it's because I have on long sleeves and I don't want to take the time to push the sleeve up. . . . But that wasn't it. I wanted to go to therapy and say, "See, Dr. Hodges? This is how much it hurts, and if you can understand that cutting yourself hurts you then maybe you can understand that what's inside you hurts even more." And once I explained that to him, I was able to stop cutting my hands.

  • • •

  Barbara: Inquire about what is going on: "Why are you cutting? What are your cuts saying? It looks like . . . you are trying to communicate something. Can you communicate it in words?"

- *Leaving the client in control in therapy.*

  This means that a therapist does not threaten to hospitalize a client against her will because of self-injury; invites her to set the pace of therapy; listens, observes, keeps track, and asks pertinent questions, but does not presume to know answers; and helps her intervene in her own self-injury process (when she is ready) by helping her explore the origins and functions of her self-injury and possible alternatives. Such control in therapy may help a client regain a sense of control over her actions and her life.[15]

Elizabeth: Instead of threatening hospitalization, let your client talk openly about what it was like for her, why she did it, and what was going on before and after. Let her feel that she is going to take control of the situation, not that you are going to take control. The client needs to feel that she is in control all the time because for a person who was abused, control is a real important thing.

• *Being informed and willing to continue learning.*

Rosa: If it's something that you're not familiar with, say so, or try to find out more. The therapist I saw a few years ago was very good in helping me deal with coming out as a lesbian, but when it came to this stuff—personally I can't do this talking to chairs and switching roles. I think that is kind of silly. She wanted me to do that and I said no. . . . I didn't feel like she understood and I actually felt a little shame, and I don't think therapists should make their patients feel ashamed.

• • •

Mary: I think they should be better versed . . . [and] treat everybody individually. I think doctors sometimes have a tendency to . . . go to a seminar and come back and [say], "This is the best way of treatment," and maybe it is but maybe it isn't for you.

• *Being compassionate.*

Erica: It's a coping mechanism; it's a survival mechanism; it's a mechanism that worked very well for a number of years. And the part that that fills in my life or another woman's life can't be given up. It's not a matter of just saying: "I'm going to stop doing this." It's a matter of leaving behind the places that made you have to do it.

• *Listening with an open mind.*

Elizabeth: I would go to my counselor thinking, "Well, at least I have my counselor to talk to and share with her." And I would go to her and say, "I was having a hard time and I cut myself." And she would say, "Oh, do you need to be in the hospital?" I'd get so angry with her: "You're not listening to me. I just shared something with you. There's obviously something wrong and I cut myself."

• *Honestly expressing her or his own feelings about self-injury.*

Jessica: I have had too many professionals who take it as an insult: "This is something you are doing *to me*" rather than "This is something you are doing and it bothers me and I need to deal with my feelings."

• • •

Esther: I think that [professionals] should be honest with the client about their own feelings. I think if they don't want to deal with someone who self-injures, they should say so because it's important that care can be there when you need it.

• *Remaining calm and kind in the face of fresh injuries.*

Elizabeth: I wanted my therapist not to get angry with me, to pay attention to the fact that something was wrong, and help me to find out what was wrong since I wasn't in touch with my feelings. When a therapist gets angry, the client feels like she has no outlet. A few times, my therapist got really upset with me when I cut, and I would leave there feeling so ashamed that I'd go home and cut again.

· · ·

Karen: Overreacting or getting excited about it [doesn't help]. . . . I just need to be nurtured when it happens and feel protected, not questioned or examined impersonally the way hospitals do if they don't have a relationship with me and are stitching me up.

• *Gently inviting discussion of self-injury.*

Peggy: Treat it like other symptoms of the trauma, as opposed to some sort of taboo. Sometimes I have a hard time talking to my therapist about stuff unless she asks me . . . because *I'm* so embarrassed about it I assume that she doesn't want to hear about it. Sometimes I think, "She doesn't really want to hear this; this isn't something she wants to deal with today." Yet, if she asks about it, then I feel like that's an invitation. She's not forcing me to tell her, just inviting me.

· · ·

Sarah O.: For the past five years I've had good therapists, and it's made the world of difference. I have a hard time with self-hate and shame. I'm not a person who likes to talk about things or admit that things affect me. One of the most helpful things for me is having my therapist ask questions or make subjects okay to talk about.

· · · · · · · · ·

Many of these women's suggestions seem to be present in Meredith's description of her own therapists. For eighteen months Meredith had both individual therapy and a "generic" therapy group for women three times weekly, then both therapies once weekly for six months. Meredith considers her past and current therapists extraordinarily gifted. She describes the beneficial things her therapists did or said, and serendipitous occurrences in her therapy that have helped enable her to curtail self-cutting:

. . . .

I was in intense therapy, and the combination of group and individual was incredibly helpful. [The two therapists] . . . have very different styles and they complemented each other well. . . . The faulty cognitions and the cloudy thinking was done with Anna in group, and the feeling stuff was done with Linda in individual. . . . Before working with [Anna], I never knew that I was smart. And I think probably one of the most important things that I have taken from my work with her is a belief in my intelligence and competence. . . .

[What makes my two therapists so good?] They have always been willing to talk with me about whatever I needed to talk about. They have allowed me to be angry with them and to talk with them about it. They have never judged me; they've never told me what to do [or] that I need to take their advice. They've always listened to me, supported me, [and] made time for me whether that means an extra appointment or an extra phone call, or accommodating my schedule which, at times, is very hectic. They've always been honest with me [and] accepted me for who I am — and they both care about me and that's something that's really new for me. . . .

They've always encouraged me not to [cut myself] and they've taught me new ways to be able to deal with things so that I wouldn't have to do it. But they've never said that I couldn't do it or that it was bad. I think that's really important. They've never judged me or shamed me for doing it. I never felt like I was on display . . . [or] like I was being *studied*. . . . It's been important for me that they've let me talk about it when I feel like I need to and they've been willing to listen to what I have to say about it — and a lot of times that's not very pleasant, it gets really graphic. And if I have gone back to doing it after a while of not doing it, it's not a shameful thing. Like, I told Linda today that I cut myself and the only thing she said to me about it was, "Can we make a safety contract for next week?" So, it wasn't looked down upon; she wasn't frustrated. She just accepts that this is how I know how to do it and that I work very hard to try to learn other ways, but sometimes the other ways aren't going to work — at least yet.

[I want to tell you] what it is that I do in my therapy that makes me be able to not cut and what are the issues that make me want to cut. I've been working individually with the same woman for over three years and think that one of the biggest things that my work with her does is it allows me to feel connected with someone. And I have found that at times I'm able to replace the cutting with my connection with her and my feeling of trust and safety with her. One time we hadn't seen each other for a while and I didn't feel a connection with her anymore. That's when I started cutting after I had been not cutting for fourteen months. I think that's why safety contracts work for me, because if I give my word to her that I won't cut myself, her trust that I will keep my word and my relationship with her is more important to me and does more for me than my cutting does. I never thought that there would be something that would be able to replace that . . . [or] serve as powerful a function in my life as the cutting does. . . . I've never been in a relationship with someone where I felt safe or where I felt like I could trust them. . . . [What makes her seem trustworthy is that] she's very gentle, kind, and compassionate, has always made time for me . . . [and] has never labeled me because of what I do or because of the things that I tell her.

[She's] teaching me how to talk about how I feel: talk it out, don't act it out. She's teaching me how to be a person, and I haven't known how to do that before, haven't known how to have feelings before and let that be okay. She taught me about acceptance, because she's very accepting of what it is I have to say. . . . I kind of functioned on automatic pilot and now I'm learning how to be human. It's scary and it's hard but I'm very lucky that I have an incredible woman sitting alongside of me as I do this.

And I have put her through *so much* — not on a conscious level — but I constantly tested her to make sure she was safe; it took me about two years before I could say I trusted her. And we just very recently began talking about the sexual abuse and my past. . . . It's taken me three years to get to the point where I feel okay enough with her to be able to talk to her about some things. So, it's been a long, grueling process for the both of us.

A really big issue for me is caring: people caring about me and me caring about other people, and me wanting other people to care about me. It's never been okay with me that I've wanted someone to care about me, and it's been incredibly painful to me when someone does care about me. And again this is the first relationship that I've been in with someone where it feels okay; it feels good. It's comforting to me to know that she cares about me: to know that I can talk with her about what's going on inside my head and how I feel about it, and to know that she's going to listen, she's going to care, she's not going to tell me not to feel that way and that it's ridiculous or anything like that. She's just going to sit there and listen.

· · · · · · · · · ·

Meredith sought help from professionals and had the good fortune to find two with the attributes she considers essential. The attributes Meredith describes in her therapists can double as guidelines for other therapists who want to know how they can better help self-injuring women and for self-injuring women who are uncertain what to look for in a therapist. Meredith's therapists care about her as a person and show it. "Caring" for someone can mean many things, but ideally it includes wanting the best for a person and helping her, when possible, achieve the best; being interested in her words and actions; and respecting her as an autonomous person. Part of the way Mcredith's therapists show their care is by being available when she needs them, a crucial and often demanding process. They do not judge her behavior, call it "sick" or "abnormal," or view it through the lens of a diagnostic label. They show respect for her autonomy by not exerting power over her through commands or threats of hospitalization. Because of her therapists' ability to understand, respect, and care, Meredith has found that a relationship can be more important and more helpful than self-cutting.

8 Sarah O.'s Past and Present

I *HATE* DOING these kind of interviews with people because it makes me seem like such a freak. I'm *not* a freak: I actually live an everyday life. I'm not a compulsive liar, I'm not a weirdo, I go to school, I'm trying to have goals, I'm sober, I have some perspective on things that have happened. . . . I guess what I'm saying is: I hope you don't get the wrong impression about who I am.

I'm a full-time student and have three part-time jobs. . . . I keep myself as busy as humanly possible so that I don't have time to sit still and deal with me. I don't do well having time on my hands; I guess it gives me too much time to think. My girlfriend always says, "Why don't you just sit on the couch and relax?" That's like torture . . . and that's when I'll [want to] self-injure.

[I stopped injuring myself about three years ago when I was twenty-four, but] for me it's very addictive. There's not too many days that go by that I don't think about doing it. It's like an obsession for me, like drinking or doing drugs. . . . The feeling is like an intense ache, a physical longing or aching to hurt myself. My arms will ache, or my whole body; I'll feel like I could crawl out of my skin, wish that I could get out of my body. I have periods of relief where I won't obsess about it — mostly, I think, because of Alcoholics Anonymous. I'm in the program, so I have tools to combat obsessions and compulsions, and I've learned other tools to use in place of any self-destructive behavior like alcohol, drugs, cutting, working-out compulsively — whatever you want to do to not feel. . . . Except, it doesn't work so well with food.

Food's kind of in a category by itself, because you don't *need* to cut yourself [or] do drugs and alcohol on an everyday basis to survive, but you have to eat. So it's always in your face; you can't avoid looking at food. I eat compulsively; I use food as my substitute drug to not feel. When I overeat or eat to the point where I'm sick, it takes away any affect that I didn't want to deal with. . . .

I'm the thinnest person in my family; they're all obese. My family medicates with food: if anything is wrong, you eat; if anything's not wrong you eat; if it's sunny you eat; if it's raining you eat. "Just keep eating and it'll be okay": that's kind of my family's motto. My whole family is extremely overweight. . . . We're all binge-eaters. . . . Food is a big problem in my family and it's obviously a huge issue in my life. It feels very uncontrollable.

I would love to be anorexic or even bulimic but I have a great aversion to vomiting. So I will never be bulimic or anorexic, but I've gone on some pretty strange crash diets where I just won't eat. When I was in college I only ate on Tuesdays and Fridays. . . . And when I ate on Tuesdays and Fridays, I would start eating first thing in the morning and I did not stop all day. I would pretty much eat enough on Tuesdays and Fridays to make up for what I didn't eat the rest of the days of the week. I binge all the time but I don't purge, so instead I'll make myself run five miles or I'll go to the gym for two hours, or I won't eat the next day, or whatever I have to do so that I won't gain weight. I'm *constantly* obsessed with my weight and my eating. If I'm not eating, I'm thinking about what I'm going to eat; and if I'm not thinking about what I'm going to eat, I'm thinking about what I just ate: everything in my life centers around food. I'm a black-and-white person and it's hard to be so extreme with food. I either eat everything or I eat nothing, and once I start eating, I'm going to eat everything.

I hate my body; . . . I'd rather hack parts of it off. . . . I've always felt very ashamed of my body. I look at everybody else and think, "Ah, if only I looked like that." I know that no matter how I looked I would hate myself, but it's always nice to think if I had somebody else's body I would feel better about it. I pretty much hate it all; there's not a whole lot about my body that I like. I don't like people looking at my body; I don't like having things go wrong with my body. I do not give my body permission to be sick or to be hurt, and I feel very betrayed when anything goes wrong with it. . . . I'm not unclean, I shower at least once or twice a day, but I don't do my nails or anything like that [and] I don't look at [my body]. Just as long as I'm clean, I don't care. . . . Going to the gym is helping my perception of my body—the way I think about myself—but it hasn't gotten manageable at all. . . .

Memories and feelings come back up, and when that happens I find my behaviors getting out of control. I have to try to figure out what is going on and work through it. I don't think that anybody goes through the healing process one time—if they do, they're pretty fortunate. You keep dealing with trauma on different levels. Things do get better but it doesn't mean that it's over, [or] that it didn't happen, [or that] it's not a part of who you are, or that it doesn't affect you in a million different ways. I believe that nine times out of ten there is a reason why I do what I do. Usually for me the behaviors are a way to avoid feeling, and usually the feeling is something connected to my past. So a lot of times I'll have to go back and try to figure out why I'm feeling upset. I'll feel sad or angry—those are probably the two main feelings that I don't want to deal with. I will sit down and try to look at where those feelings are coming from and talk about them or do whatever I need to do with them. If I can get through the feeling I can usually stop the behavior. [Otherwise], I'll start using destructive behaviors to not deal with my emotions. . . . With my drug and alcohol use, the obsession to drink and use drugs has been lifted. But, I think that with each behavior you have to go through the same things over and over again until you master it. So I think I'll be here for a while.

When I was younger, I did different things. I didn't start cutting right away. When I was a kid, I did many less obvious things. Like, I broke many of my fingers in doors unintentionally: I would forget to take my hand out of the door. Then I was like, "Oh, maybe I could break my fingers again. I've done it before, by accident, so if I did it again it would seem like an accident." I used to bang them with hammers or other blunt instruments to try to break my fingers—which I never succeeded at doing. I think that started at the end of sixth grade; I would have been about eleven. I punch[ed] walls for a while; that pretty much stopped when I almost broke my knuckles. I liked to bang my head, . . . but not to the point of giving myself a concussion. [But] I mainly used cutting. . . . I've tried to stop pretty much all my self-injurious behaviors, [but] I still do food [and] compulsive exercising.

I don't remember why the self-injury started. When I was younger and the behaviors first started, it was more out of a feeling of not being real, like I felt fake or inhuman, I didn't feel or I felt numb, and that's why I would cut: to feel something. As I got older, a lot of times anger would precipitate cutting. . . . For me, rage and anger are very physical sensations. . . . All the physiological things happen: my heart rate increases, my adrenaline begins pumping . . . my jaw clenches, I shake. You know the saying you "see red"? I almost see red: literally rage changes my visual perceptions. And I feel very out of control and very on the edge of totally losing control—on the edge of actually saying or doing something that would be hurtful to others. Sometimes I'll feel like I'm on the edge of going insane—not being able to come back from wherever I am headed. I don't like to be out of control; I don't like to feel anger. For me, anything is preferable to feeling angry. I hate rage, and I think that's a big part of why rage is so dangerous for me. The more angry and rageful I get, the more I hate myself; and the more I hate myself, the more angry I feel. Rage feels very evil to me; I don't like it because that's not how I want to be. When I'm rageful, I have a really hard time controlling my behavior. I've gotten a lot better with it—I have to practice feeling rage and not acting on it. And I wasn't very good at not acting on [it]. . . . I think that's why rage made me feel so evil because I feel hateful and angry, like I want to do physical and emotional harm to anyone who's near me. It's not a pleasant feeling. . . .

Because I can't deal with anger a lot of times, immediately I start thinking, "I hate myself, I have to punish myself." I think that not feeling those physical sensations and getting angry with myself is part of the body sensation that I feel—I don't know if that makes sense. Instead of feeling them as anger at what I was angry at, they start to feel more like an ache in my body to cut myself. Instead of feeling angry at everybody else, I'll start to think to myself, "Well, it's really me that I'm angry at; I'm really the idiot." Then I start to get mad at myself, and the more I get mad at myself, the more I feel like I need to cut my body—the more my body actually *hurts* for a release. Instead of shaking and being so angry I could punch something else, I turn it around and I start to ache to hurt myself.

I don't know what to do with the desire to cut myself once I feel that way. It feels like the only thing I can do once I'm there is some kind of physical damage to myself. I need to release the anger somehow, and you can tell me to bang the pillows on my bed as much as you want but it just doesn't do the trick. Today, the best thing for me to do is to work out, take a shower—stuff like that. But it's still not nearly as effective as cutting myself: cutting really does the trick quick.

A lot of things have happened to me. My father's done a lot of really hurtful things, and I can't be angry with him because, you know, he's just an alcoholic; he's the same as me. I have a hard time being angry with him. It's like, "Yeah, it was kind of a bad thing that he did, but I can't get mad at him. He's just a sick person." I guess I've gone around in circles with anger. It's much easier to hate yourself than it is to hate other people. There are situations in which you can't pin it on anybody; there's just no one else to blame. If you can't blame a specific person then you can blame life, and life would ultimately be God's responsibility, so you blame God. Then you decide that there's no God, and who else is there [to blame] but yourself?

Of all the horrible things I could do to myself, cutting is definitely my favorite. It doesn't cost much; it's also very easy to hide as long as you don't get too out of control and [then] do it in places where people can see it. Drugs and alcohol are much more perceivable. Food's very accessible but getting fat just makes the whole thing worse, so you don't want to use food too much. With cutting, there's also a tremendous sense of relief: the body automatically starts producing chemicals that make you feel better. [Also], you actually have something you can see and say, "Oh, this would cause pain; this is a reason why I hurt. I don't understand other reasons why I hurt, but this I can see; this is a legitimate reason to feel pain." It's much easier to experience pain because of something tangible, as opposed to feeling emotional pain and not understanding why. I think that I was also cutting to punish myself. I would feel dirty or disgusting, and cutting was sort of a punishment. I guess I was trying to cleanse myself.

Blood is very gratifying—I don't really know [why]. I guess because it's very real: blood is what makes me alive—I *am* alive, I *am* like other people. There's something very—I don't want to say "cathartic," but maybe it is—about letting blood come out of you. It's like, "Ah, this is relief." It's also something to watch, something to occupy my attention, you know; manipulating my blood once it's out of my body helps me to focus and calm down. [So, for all those reasons, cutting is] preferable to other things.

I definitely like blood: seeing my blood, playing with my blood, and all those sort of gruesome, disgusting things I can do. I started with the breaking of the fingers because it was something that I had learned. I didn't know that I could cut myself: I was still young and hadn't yet figured it out. So, I achieved something better when I found out that I could cut myself. . . . I'd say I was probably around twelve or thirteen. That isn't to say that I stopped doing other things, but I started to realize that cutting was much more fun. . . . It was like, "Oh, *this* is really what I wanted."

I enjoy watching my blood flow. A lot of times I would cut myself and watch the path that it traveled over my body as it left, and collect it in a bucket. I would touch it; get it on my fingers, feel its consistency—this is kind of disgusting—it's kind of a weird texture, sticky. Sometimes I would get worried that it wasn't real because you don't expect blood to be sticky. I would play around with it and then start to worry that it wasn't real, that I wasn't real again. Then I would have to cut more to make sure that it was actually blood. So sometimes it wasn't all that helpful. [Sometimes I would have to taste it.] I wouldn't consume great quantities of it, but I had to make sure that it wasn't fake or it wasn't just red-colored water. I worried that maybe I wasn't real, so I decided to use whatever methods I had to make sure that I was real. I liked playing with my blood. I would use it like it was finger paint. I was mesmerized by it. Probably by the time I got to that point, unless I was starting to panic that it wasn't real, I was pretty happy, pretty numb, so playing with the blood was more like something to do; it was gratifying and fulfilling. It was something that focused me; took my attention away from everything else. [If I had used paint,] it wouldn't have done it for me. . . .

Can I trace [self-injury] back to any physical event or situation that happened? No, I think it more or less came out of a need to escape feelings. I don't think there was one event. In general, I was unable to deal with feelings [and] I definitely came up with the behaviors to suit what I needed. Sure [I know where the feelings came from]. I don't think that I had the greatest time growing up. I had kind of a strange childhood—I mean a lot of people

have; I don't think it was worse for me than it was for a lot of people. . . .
My father's an alcoholic; he was physically and emotionally abusive to my
mother and me. There [were] some happy times, but in general I remember
getting beaten a lot and once he tried to kidnap me. My mom stayed with
him for thirteen years; she probably suffered from battered wife syndrome,
whatever they call that these days. I spent some time in police stations writing up reports of abuse. I grew up in a farming community, so [my mother
and I] used to run to my aunt's house and she would grab the shotgun and
stand by the front door in case he came after us. I spent a lot of time living
with my aunt because my parents were separated a lot or they didn't want me
around because they were having trouble. I think a lot of that was just my
mom wanting to get me out of the situation physically. This is speculation,
but I had spinal meningitis when I was a kid and the doctors never knew
why. When I was twenty, they found that I had a cerebral spinal fluid leak
from some kind of head trauma or birth defect. And at first I was like, "Oh,
it's a birth defect," but now I believe it was more likely that I got hit in the
head one too many times. That was my father's favorite place to hit me. My
younger cousin told me that there was a time when my father hit me in the
head so hard I passed out. I don't want to make him seem like an animal, and
I don't know if it's true, but it would make sense that he caused the crack in
my head.

   My father's big thing was that he would hit me once and I would cry, then
he would say, "Stop crying or I'll really give you something to cry about." It
used to escalate. I could tell he didn't *want* to hit me—I knew he didn't. So
he would just keep saying that and hitting me, trying to get me to stop crying.
I think it's probably very similar to cutting. It's like, you make a mistake and
you do something, then you're really angry at yourself for doing it, so you
keep doing it because you're so mad. *I* do this; that's why I can understand
why he did it. I don't go around hitting people, but I do other things. Like I'll
get so mad at myself for doing something that I'll cut myself. Today, instead
of cutting, I use food. I'll overeat and then get so angry at myself I'll continue
to eat more.

   And then, on the other hand, I was in a sexual relationship [from the age
of four with] my older cousin Jim. It started out innocently, like, "What does
your anatomy look like?" You know, pulling down your pants, seeing what
things looked like. It was more that he wanted to know what I looked like. I
was upset about it, but I didn't necessarily feel like, "This is really *wrong!*" I
don't think I had a sense that it was wrong until he started saying stuff like,
"You can never tell. We can't let anybody else know." Until [then], I don't
really know if I had a clue that what was happening was as devastating as it

was. There was always something secretive about it, so I knew that there was something wrong and I knew that I didn't feel all that great about it. But I didn't really realize where it was going. It didn't stop there, and it actually lasted until I was eighteen. [When] I was twelve, it got to the point of penetration. I never stopped it; I was never the kind of person who could say no. I was never physically forced to do anything with Jim. I think it was more or less that I didn't want to disappoint him. He was the only person who spent time with me. I felt like I was as much to blame for the situation [as he was]: I couldn't say no.

I think until probably my mid-teens, the pleasure was purely that Jim would spend time with me. The emotional care that I got when I was with him was something that I needed. Because after the sexual act happened, we would hang out: we would go for a walk in the woods, and when I got older, we would get stoned together. So I think the pleasure that I felt was more of companionship, and I felt close to him when I was growing up. . . . I guess I felt that Jim and I had that sort of relationship where I would not be able to go on without him — that he was the only person I could relate to, who understood me, who knew how I felt. . . .

My whole family's pretty sick, and the abuse that's taken place in my life is not the first time; [it's part of] a generational cycle of abuse. So, I always felt bad for Jim, for both of us. I had a lot of pity for my whole family; they were really stuck. I felt that with Jim, we could transcend our family and make it out. At the time, I couldn't *name* any of it; I didn't understand any of it.

I'm not sure I would [say that Jim seduced me]. By the time I was a freshman in high school, I got really low. I was active with my drug and alcohol addiction, I was reading a lot of existentialist stuff, I had pretty much checked out of life. I had decided that I didn't give a shit about most anything. At that point I actually started seeking him out because I had nothing. There weren't a lot of people around for me. My mom [had] divorced my father and remarried. She was working two jobs and putting herself through school because my father refused to pay child support. . . . I didn't care for my stepfather. So there weren't a lot of people around. I still *looked* okay. I was leading this double life: I was getting A's in school, playing three varsity sports, working part-time at my uncle's restaurant — I was doing all these wonderful things and on the inside I was dying. I could never let anybody know that except Jim. And I wouldn't say, "I feel like I'm going to kill myself today," but I would do what he wanted me to do just to be with someone. By that time, I think he was actually pulling back: I don't think that he wanted to continue what we were doing. But I started seeking him out because I still needed somebody. One of the hardest things for me today is to forgive myself for not ending the relationship. The longer I let it go on, the more I hated myself. I had pretty much set myself up by that point, . . . I feel like I had stopped caring.

By the time I was in seventh grade, I wanted to die. I started doing a lot of acting out, I started cutting, I started spending a lot of time just thinking that I'd rather be dead, and I started having actual plans of suicide. I couldn't afford to care anymore. I felt like every time I cared, I got disappointed. I started not to worry about what I was doing; I started enjoying self-destructive behavior. The more I decided that I didn't care, the more trouble I got myself into.

I'm also gay, so I had all of that to deal with. When I hit puberty I started realizing that I wasn't the same as everybody else. . . . I felt intense pressure to try to be straight, which I did all through high school. I started to learn what "gay" was when I was in the seventh and eighth grade[s], and I do believe that I knew inside that I was, but I could never admit it to my conscious mind — it was horrible. I come from a very small hick town. Everybody's the same; they're all lower to middle class families, not poor, but certainly not doing all that great. . . . There was just no one who was different. When I was in seventh grade, a couple of people in senior class were accused of being gay — in fact they were gay, and they were tormented because of it. So, I learned early on that it was *not* okay to be gay. You would rather be anything else in the world besides gay, and if you were gay, you were doomed to that sort of persecution all your life. So I pretty much decided that I would not be gay, and I tried that for six years. I'm sure that had a lot to do with my hating myself, hating my body. It was a huge relief when I came out at eighteen.

During junior high school, I started to feel really, *really* different. I worried that I wasn't human — I worried that I was evil. It was unspoken until I was about fifteen or so, but my family has a lot of ritualistic abuse which happened to my mother and her sisters. So, there were a lot of satanic undertones to everything. In fact, my mother was told by her parents that I would be the devil's baby. It was never spoken, but I kind of feel like I was brought up that way. My mother was always really, really afraid that something bad was going to happen to me. My grandparents told her that I would die, and that if I survived, I was the devil's child. . . . There were some very evil places on our property where we didn't go. You didn't know why you didn't go, but you didn't go. There were burial sites that smelled foul from mass sacrifices, I guess, that my grandparents used to have, or something — something really weird. And Jim and I knew about them; we knew that there was something really evil there, but we didn't know what it was. We used to make fun of it, like kids do, and try to concoct stories about what it was.

If I had to say what precipitated [cutting] at that point, it wasn't so much anger as feeling different. I felt like I was watching myself in a movie — that this couldn't be me; that life had to be more than this; and if this was what life was, I didn't want any part of it. A lot of times I used it to feel like I had some control: that if I wanted to kill myself, I could; that suicide was always an option for me; that I didn't need life. [It was] a way to protect myself, like, "Yeah, I'll live today, but I don't *have* to. If I decide I don't want to, I don't have to." I guess there was a lot of anger going on, but I *could not* get angry to save my life.

In high school, people mostly stayed away from me. I was kind of an odd-ball; people saw me as pretty much weird, disturbed — a loser, a loner. I had a lot of acquaintances; I didn't have a whole lot of friends. I kind of fit in everywhere and nowhere at once. I could hang out with people who got straight A's because I got straight A's; I could hang out with the jocks because I played sports; I could hang out with the band people because I played in the band; I could hang out with the losers because I did drugs; I could hang out anywhere I wanted, but I didn't fit in anywhere. I think a lot of people knew that I was gay although it wasn't said or acknowledged, and certainly it wasn't said or acknowledged by me. People didn't talk to me a lot. People didn't know how to deal with me; they didn't know how to take me; they didn't know how to help me. So the way that my entire community — school, family, every-body — dealt with it was to not ask because they had no clue what to do. I think I scared them.

When I was in eighth grade, I really needed help and no one was noticing me. I couldn't ask for help myself because I was leading this double life where everything was "fine": I was doing really well in school, I was active in sports and music — and I was dying inside. I didn't know how to ask for help, and I didn't really believe that there was anything that could help me. I felt so responsible for my situation: I believed that it was my fault and that I didn't have the right to ask for help. I had already been cutting for a while, and I don't remember how it started, but I started cutting in public: I did it on the school bus on the way home. It started to get really convenient be-cause I was starting to do cocaine and I always had a razor blade on me to cut cocaine. I was sitting alone with a nice, clean, shiny razor blade. Although I couldn't admit it at the time, looking back I think it must have been that I needed attention. I needed somebody to ask me what was wrong; I needed somebody to help me, yet I couldn't ask for help. It was an obsession — I mean, I could not be left alone with a razor blade; it was like putting a bottle of Jack Daniels in front of an alcoholic. I wasn't really cutting at that point, I was kind of scratching or etching little things into my arm . . . or carving words into my body, taking my time, being meticulous to detail. "Die," "death," "the end" were recurring words. "Die," that was a big theme. Now I can say that I didn't want to die, but at that time I didn't know that I didn't want to.

No one noticed that I was cutting. I wore long sleeves a lot and the few who did see never asked or said anything. I don't know what they were thinking. . . . Oh God, I think about how blatant it was. . . . Like in physical education in high school, I walked around with medical tape on my arms to hide the cuts and no one said anything. I was doing cocaine in classes with some of my friends, and I would carve into my arms with a razor blade while we were in class, and no one said anything. . . . I can think of at least three teachers who must have noticed, especially the phys ed teachers. . . . I know that one of them saw me putting [the medical tapes] on; I know that they saw the cuts, but they never said anything.

My friends [finally] went to the band director and told him that I was cutting myself, and he's the one who sent me to the school psychologist. But she was no help. . . . She didn't ask me about the cutting; she didn't ask me about much of anything that I can remember. . . . To be honest, I thought she was an idiot and I wasn't about to tell her anything. I guess the biggest problem with me was that I was so good at putting things into little compartments and sealing them up. I had no idea how much things were affecting me, and I didn't want to believe that they were.

Also, I was doing cocaine in public. It amazes me how long I kept doing this before anybody found out. It was well over a year before anybody asked me about it. It wasn't like people didn't see me doing cocaine. A group of students would pass around one of those little pocket-sized mirrors with cocaine on it during classes. I was screaming for somebody to say something, and no one would. Eventually one of the kids on the school bus saw me etching something into my arm and told his parents, and his parents called the school. I guess they finally got enough complaints about me doing all these kind of heinous things. By the time I was a sophomore in high school, this all came out and I was hospitalized.

At that point, no one knew what my drug intake was or how much I was cutting myself, or if I had done any physical damage to my body by using drugs and alcohol. So, they put me in a regular hospital on the psychiatric unit for an evaluation. They "determined" that I was borderline personality, and their recommendation was that I needed long-term psychiatric care. I was introduced to AA, and I opted to go to a drug rehab because after sitting in a hospital for a while, I knew that I needed help, and this was my opportunity. So I went through drug rehab . . . for four and a half months. [Then] their recommendation was that I do a two-year inpatient psych-unit program. I opted not to because I thought I was going to die before I graduated high school. I wanted to live the rest of my high school days before I died. . . . So I went back to school; I stayed sober; I pretty much stopped the cutting behavior or at least if I did it, it was secretive and more controlled. I was able to maintain some control for five years. I got into a relationship with a woman. She kind of held me together for another four and a half or five years and then she left me . . . because we had been having problems in the relationship, especially around sex, which is a recurring theme in my relationships. So she went and slept with someone else.

My worst cutting episode happened just before I graduated from college. I had no idea what I was doing with my life; I didn't feel competent teaching, which is what my degree is in; and I was working at a stupid job. My girlfriend left me, and after that, all of my past issues started to surface. I was living alone and keeping odd hours: I used to work from one in the afternoon to one in the morning. I had no friends; I wasn't doing anything besides going to work, coming home, staying up all night watching cable, and then getting up in time to go to work again. I was depressed; I was eating, living, sleeping, breathing sexual abuse. I finally just lost it. I don't remember how the cutting spree started but I remember being in the middle of it, and being like, "Wow, this is cool." Then I remember towards the end getting worried; I was thinking that maybe it would be good to kill myself. Once I start on a spree like that, it puts me in a separate reality. Things like killing yourself become more of an option and seem a lot easier to actually achieve. When I tried to go really hard and slash myself I would close my eyes: it's kind of a reflex. So I kept trying to practice to see if I could keep my eyes open. I was pissed off that I couldn't keep my eyes open. I started getting into a lot of slashing, seeing if I could keep my eyes open while I slashed myself deeper and deeper; or cutting the same cut many times over to see how deep I could get it. . . .

I [finally] drove myself [to the hospital] because I was really out of control. It wasn't—I mean, I say that I want to die, but I don't really think I want to die. I think I just didn't want to live the way I was living; I didn't want to feel what I was feeling; I [wanted to] be somebody else. So, when I get out of control cutting, I start to get worried that I—you know, I do have the capability, I do have the anger to kill myself: I'm that mad at myself that I could. But I don't really want to; I would rather learn how to live differently.

[But let me go back a bit to explain]. . . . When I was growing up, between sixth and seventh grade, when I left grammar school and went to high school, everything changed for me. . . . Starting in May, this awesome dread [of everything] came over me, and I just never got out from underneath it, my whole life. I was kind of paralyzed with fear for a while. That's when I started to realize that I was going to die. And from that time on I never believed that I would live very long. From around the end of sixth grade, I believed I was going to die at eighteen. And when I didn't die at eighteen, I was kind of upset about it; I felt betrayed. Then I figured I had miscalculated. I figured, "Oh, it must have been nineteen, nineteen, right, right, right." And then I turned nineteen and I was like, "Well, now what's going on?" and I got more and more angry. And then when I turned twenty, I thought, "Well, certainly I'm not going to turn twenty-one!" And then I had that brain surgery and I really believed that that was it. I believed, "Alright, I finally got it right. I'm going to die now and that's the way it was supposed to be. I just made a mistake in calculating: it was twenty, it wasn't eighteen." Then I lived through the surgery, and that was like the beginning of the end for me. When I lived through that surgery I started to realize that I wasn't going to die. I started to get really mad at God because — not that I really believed in God anymore — but I figured that he had screwed me enough, and I thought, "Well, he had an opportunity to kill me and he didn't." And I felt betrayed. I was like, "You fucker! You put me through all this; you could be merciful." I had a lot of friends die during high school and I thought that that was better; I thought that they got off easy. . . . I started to feel . . . tortured, and I also had to face up to the fact that a lot of the stuff that my father had done did affect me. No matter how much I didn't want to be angry with him, I had to admit that it affected me. . . .

Up until that point, my trumpet was saving my life. I was a music major, and I played the trumpet from the time I was in sixth grade up until my junior [year] in college. . . . It was the only way that I could express myself. When I was a freshman in college I was playing about five or six hours a day just practicing; that's not including the ensembles that I played in. The trumpet was the most important thing to me. I believed that I wanted to be cremated and have my ashes put inside my trumpet and buried that way. [Then] I found out that I had to have the [brain] surgery done because the pressure of playing the trumpet was making the cerebral spinal fluid leak worse. I had to stop playing; . . . then I couldn't play for six months after the surgery. So I didn't pick up the trumpet again until the following spring. I was so frustrated that everything I had worked for was shot. Playing a musical instrument that involves muscles in your face, you have to work at it and practice it and get [the muscles] back. [But] I have a very black-and-white attitude, you know; I'm not one to say, "Oh well, I'll just practice for a couple of months and get it back." I'll be like, "It's ruined now; I'll never have it again." And also I think that whole time was really emotional for me — it just got a little too painful; I got to the point where I couldn't handle my feelings. I couldn't manipulate my trumpet the way I wanted to, and it ruined it for me. I think to a large degree, not playing my trumpet made it a lot easier to self-injure. I think that playing my trumpet was a release, was a way of expressing myself, and when I didn't have it, I turned to self-injury once again. So I think not having that was really hard. I still haven't gotten it back; it's something that plagues me to this day. Currently a goal in my therapy is to be able to play the trumpet again. Right now, it's really a sore spot. Not a day goes by [that I don't think], "Wow, I walked away from it!" I haven't touched my trumpet in three years, and this is something that I did five or six hours a day for twelve or thirteen years. And I just walked away. . . .

I've been in a good way for a couple of years: I've been starting to live my life, starting to enjoy my life. Every once in a while some dirt gets kicked up or something will get set off in me that makes me start thinking about things in a negative way. My thinking goes first; and as soon as my thinking goes, my affect goes; and as soon as my affect goes, I say, "Uh oh! Got to do something not to feel this." It doesn't matter to me if it's feeling like a failure, or feeling angry — because feeling angry for me *is* feeling like a failure, for some reason. A lot of times I'll feel like I'm acting a movie, like this just can't be my life. You know, I had such different notions of who I would be and what I would be than what I've turned out to be. Now I'm realizing that I have more choice and more say about how I want my life to be and I can change it more; I'm more effective at directing where I'm going. But when I start to feel like, "This isn't how it's supposed to be," I think that's a lot of what precipitates feelings of cutting or doing other self-injurious behavior.

I have a really hard time with getting tense and anxious and worked up, and for me, that's bordering on anger. Sometimes for me it's hard to tell when I'm just anxious and when I'm angry. I'm a hyper person anyway, not to mention that I drink a lot of caffeine. A lot of times, when I get really worked up, sports, running, working out, hauling wood, moving somebody from apartment to apartment — any kind of physical activity like that — helps me immensely. A lot of times I'll just work myself physically until I can't move because it's relief, it brings about calm and peace afterward.

I used to [injure myself] a lot at work and at school. . . . Whenever anything goes wrong, I'm very critical of myself, so usually in those situations the first thing I think about is hurting myself. I do something socially wrong at school, or I make a mistake at work, it's the first thing that comes to mind. It's just me, you know. Like, I would make a mistake, . . . at work . . . just something stupid; something socially would happen and I would feel like an idiot; I would embarrass myself; or I would put my foot in my mouth. And the first thing that would come to my mind is, "I have to go lock myself in the bathroom and cut myself; I'm such an idiot; I don't know why I just said that; I wish I hadn't done that; I hate me." I don't cut myself today, but that's the first thought through my head. It's not like I think, "Oh, well, that was just a mistake," and ten minutes later I think, "Well, I should cut myself." It's like, "I made a mistake; I wish I hadn't done that; I hate myself; go cut yourself." I think I've gotten a little better in that I'm a little more tolerant of myself, of being human, and of making mistakes. But, whenever anything goes wrong, I have to be vigilant about not letting myself think that way. I have to really stay on myself, because [hating myself and wanting to cut] is my first tendency.

I think I've been thinking wrong all my life. And it's only since I've become willing to try to think differently and try to work through issues in therapy that I've been able to become a little more tolerant of myself. You know, self-hate is one of the primary reasons why I cut. I try not to hate myself; I try to give myself a break sometimes. I struggle with that. I remember fighting with therapists because I've always believed that forgiving yourself for making mistakes was just a rationalization allowing mediocrity, . . . [and] I never wanted to be mediocre in anything. I have very low impulse control, so it takes vigilance and practice and willingness not to follow through on thoughts, and to try to say, "Okay, that's not reality, that's just my messed up thinking, that's just old tapes," or whatever. . . . If I was going to try to be tolerant with myself today, I would try to think, "I don't need to cut myself; this isn't that big of a deal," [or] "This wasn't the end of the world; I don't need to cut myself over such a stupid situation." But, it's a lot of work.

I think there's two ways to stop hurting yourself: healthy ways, and unhealthy ways. . . . Unhealthy things that I've used to not hurt myself in the past would be food: food is a major one. If I feel like cutting, I can eat a box of cookies, and usually that will put me far enough out of reality that I can either just go to sleep or it takes my mind off of it. Usually it puts me to sleep; I'll eat myself into a sugar coma or something. That's a dangerous thing to do because after I've recovered from the sugar-induced sleepiness, I hate myself that much more. It works for the moment, but it usually has rebound effects that are far worse. In fact, eating for me is my final frontier . . . that's what I'm working on right now. That is the biggest issue in my life, the one thing that can make me suicidal instantaneously: if I overeat, it's all over. I struggle with that on a daily basis. [What makes me suicidal is] just overeating, feeling fat, feeling bad about myself, hating myself. On a daily basis, I don't really hate myself a whole lot for other things. I've gotten much more tolerant with making mistakes, or putting my foot in my mouth socially — stuff like that. You know, I used to get very upset if I embarrassed myself publicly in any way. And nowadays, I just kind of laugh at myself. But if I eat a box of cookies, I can't laugh at myself. I use food a lot to alter affect, so it's a pretty dangerous game. So that is one way that I've used not to cut, but it's not a good way.

[After eating cookies and feeling worse I used to be] more likely to cut, [but] the only thing that I do today if that happens is go to the gym: that's the healthiest way that I've found not to cut. I get very, I guess, anxious; I have all this excess energy and anger or whatever — I don't even know if it's anger sometimes, it's just all this energy, like, I feel very wound up. When I get like that, whether it's self-hate, anger, feeling upset or confused, or whatever, the best way for me to get rid of that energy, instead of cutting to release it, is to go to the gym.

[At the gym] I work out regularly and I have for many years. I have a set routine: I do at least fifteen minutes if not a half-hour of cardiovascular sort of exercises, like running on a treadmill or using the bike machines. And then I lift weights [and] do sit-ups and push-ups. I work out every day at least fifty minutes, but usually about an hour and fifteen minutes to an hour and a half unless I'm really too busy, which happens very infrequently. Sometimes I'll do my regular workout in the morning, and I'll come home [in the evening] upset, like I had a bad day at school, I felt stupid, or whatever. If I just need to go to the gym to stop myself from doing unhealthy things, like overeating, or cutting, I can just run on the treadmill for twenty minutes and I'll come home and feel a million percent better. So, my daily working out . . . helps me because I feel better about myself. . . . I think it's most important for my eating, to combat poor self-esteem [about] my body. But in emergency situations where I just need to release energy or I need to take my mind off of things, running on a treadmill is fine for me. It takes my mind off of it; it wears me out. When I'm worn out, I don't care! I don't sit there and think, "Oh, I was such an idiot," or "Oh, I'm such a jerk." I'm just like, "Oh, I'm tired; I want to go to bed."

That is the best way [for me to keep from self-injuring]. . . . Some people say, "Take a shower," which I have found helpful but I've found unhelpful also: when you take a hot shower, your veins stick out, and that, for me, is not a good thing when I'm feeling like cutting. So, although it does help sometimes, it's not always the best idea. Other things are: if I can get myself involved in something, anything — which is hard to do when you're feeling really out there — but, if I can get myself into a book, if I can get myself into a computer game, or a crossword puzzle — anything that will occupy my mind so that I can't think. That's mainly what the object is: to not think or feel. . . .

I certainly couldn't just change my thinking if I wasn't doing other things. Like, if I wasn't working out every morning, I wouldn't think differently about myself. Changing the way you think isn't just like one morning you say to yourself, "Okay, I'm not going to think the same way anymore." You require some kind of action. I guess I've always felt like — how does the saying go? — "Right action will bring right thinking," but you can't get to right thinking without right action. You know, if I can just force myself to do the right thing, I will eventually think differently. Whereas, if I'm cutting, I'll never think differently. . . . At the moment, [I'm trying to act and think differently.] If something comes up, and I start to think poorly — and in a work or school situation you can't just walk out of school and go work out. So, if things come up, I can't walk out and go to the gym, but I can think, "Okay, this isn't so bad." And I think if I wasn't doing all these other things in my life, I wouldn't be able to change my thoughts like that. [By "all these other things" I don't mean just working out.] Like, I've gone to therapy for a number of years trying to work on past issues. I think if I hadn't tried to think differently about my past, that things wouldn't have changed. If I hadn't gotten out of the dead-end jobs that I was in and tried to go back to school, I don't think that my self-esteem would have gotten much better. And certainly, the jobs that I [had] also lended themselves to poor eating, poor sleeping habits, which have made a huge difference in my life, more than I ever wanted to give them credit for. Just trying to be a better person, working towards physical and spiritual growth, trying to do more for other people, stuff like that. . . .

If I want to abuse my body by cutting, I don't necessarily see anything inherently wrong with that, although it's a taboo in our society. Other people [abuse] their bodies by smoking or drinking or taking high risks by parachute jumping. But it upsets the people around me, and that's one big reason why I don't want to do it. . . . Guilt was [also] a pretty big motivating factor for me to stop cutting because I had this person who I cared very much about who I didn't want to hurt. And I think that played an important part, even if it was just guilt that kept me away from it for five minutes so that I could do something different. That was better than nothing; at least it stopped it for the moment. . . . [She was a factor in my ability to stop] and even more maybe in my ability not to do it now. Because I have built a life for myself, and for the most part I'm happy with where I am — not necessarily with where I am but my potential to reach where I want to be. I don't want to jeopardize that. And she's made it quite clear that [cutting is] not something that she could stick around for; that she does not want to be with me and watch me do that to myself. Cutting yourself is wonderful and it feels great, but it's not worth the consequences. I'm much more able to think things through today and say, "If I do this, it's going to mean this." There are consequences to my cutting; it doesn't just affect me. . . . If it did, I'd probably have to say that I would do it still. [But] it affects people around me: it upsets my family, it upsets my lover, it upsets the people that I work with. Like in my job in 1991, the people who knew that I was doing it were kind of freaked out about it. So, it's not just simply, "Sarah does this and enjoys it, and that's fine." . . .

Yes, my life has changed since I stopped self-injuring, but I think it had more to do with the reasons why I was able to stop self-injury and the changing my thinking and all that good stuff . . . that allowed me to stop cutting. It's more related to the whole picture. I think my life has changed because I have been able to deal with a lot of things that happened in the past and a lot of things about myself, and that has allowed me to stop cutting. Certainly stopping cutting helps my self-esteem; I was never very proud of cutting. . . . I'm enjoying wearing short sleeves; that's kind of nice. But other than that, stopping wasn't as important as why I was able to stop.

I've stopped hiding my scars. Especially in summertime, when it's hot, I don't wear long sleeves anymore. And when I'm wearing a tee shirt, people ask. Sometimes [I'm honest], and sometimes I'm honest only after I'm caught lying. The person that I am today doesn't want to lie, but the person that I am today doesn't want to tell. So it depends on the situation. . . .

But if you go to the gym in sleeves it's really uncomfortable. I'm embarrassed and self-conscious enough; the gym is the one place where I'm starting to feel okay. As I get more into working out and eating right, more and more I'm trying to let go of my eating problems, more and more I'm feeling better about myself. And the more I feel better about myself, the more I feel like I can't be bothered to — if I let myself feel embarrassed and ashamed of [my scars], it ruins what good I'm trying to accomplish. [So, when I work out], I wear short sleeves and shorts. Luckily, no one's asked me; . . . people kind of do their own thing there. I try to work out in areas where no one else is working out because I am self-conscious. But if they see me, I don't care. . . .

When I was sixteen, . . . they diagnosed me as being borderline. You know, I fit the criteria; you only have to fit five out of nine criteria — a lot of people could fit that. And so I was put on antipsychotics. . . . I stayed on Mellaril for a year and a half or two years, . . . and I was on Prolixin — I don't think I should have been tranquilized quite so heavily. From the way they treated me, I felt like my personality was deformed and it was irreversible. There wasn't a whole lot I felt anybody was going to do for me or that they thought they could do for me. I felt like [they thought], "Oh well; this is the way you are. It's worthless trying to work with you because you're not going to get any better." I guess I felt like the only thing that they could do was tranquilize me so that I wouldn't be a problem; so that I wouldn't act out. I was in the general psych ward. . . . When I got out of there, their recommendation was that I do a two-year locked psych unit for God knows what because no one ever asked me what was going on. No one ever asked me point blank, "Has something been going on with you sexually?" And it never came up for me. It wasn't like I had forgotten it, but I just never made the connection that there could be anything wrong. . . . It wasn't like I ever forgot my memories or repressed them or had multiple selves, I just didn't *think* about it. I didn't realize how much it was affecting me, and no one asked. . . . I made it through the mental health system seeing therapists and everything else for twelve years before I ever brought it up that something was going on. . . .

[So] one of the reasons why I'm doing this [interview] is because I feel like my experience has not been dealt with well in the mental health system. I feel like I was misdiagnosed; the treatment I was given was not effective or appropriate. Part of the reason why I want to help this effort is because I don't want other people to do the same thing. . . .

[But] I think it's also important for me to do [this interview] because by talking about things, I think, eventually things do get better—just by saying words or thinking about it in a different way. Once you say something and get it out, it feels different, it looks different, it fits together better with other things.

[It's hard to explain why saying words is important]. . . . I always thought when I was growing up that if somebody just told me what to do to feel better, like, just gave me a list [of] ten things to do, like: "Run around the block three times, do fifteen push-ups, say five Hail Marys, and whip yourself with a wet noodle, and then you'll feel better." But there was never anything tangible that somebody could say, "This is what you do to feel better—to get better." They always said, "It's a process; it takes time to process things." And I would always ask, "Well, what the hell does processing things mean?" And they were like, "You just keep talking about them." And I'm like, "Well, I don't want to keep talking about them." You know, you go around in a circle. And I think that finally after God knows how many years I've been doing this, it just happened. It *is* a process and I guess when I try to describe what it means to process things, talking comes in somewhere. I don't know why it works; I don't understand why I have to say things before I can look at them differently; I don't understand why I have to say things before they have any emotional meaning to me—I don't understand that, but that's the way it is.

9 Recovery
Hopes and Achievements

. . . .

Karen: I feel like I could recapture something that I have lost if I could stop. For one thing, I'd like my body a lot better and I'd use it and feel good about it. I'd *do* things, you know, outdoor things where you can take your clothes off, and go swimming, things like that. I just envision this *freedom* that I haven't had, especially with my kids while they're little. And also, I hurt a lot. It feels like I've always got some pain somewhere. So, I feel that if I didn't cut myself, I'd have more of a life.

. . . .

LIKE KAREN, many women who chronically injure themselves are able to envision a time when they no longer need to do so. They see a future free of self-injury in which they can feel better about themselves. The very fact that they had conquered something would give them pride, a feeling they badly need. Controlling self-injury would promote a sense of overall greater self-control, and the shame of having "given in" to self-injury would subside. Increased self-esteem might lead to further changes: a different job or career, completing a languishing project, entering a new relationship, taking a vacation. If they could stop, they would have more time and energy to devote to the ordinary concerns of life. They might regain the full use of their bodies: play on the beach, swim, wear clothes that reveal their arms and legs. They could feel that they were like other people, not "freaks" or "bizarre." They would not have to worry about tense situations or fear long meetings or workshops when release through self-injury is impossible. When no scars are fresh, they might be more honest about self-injury, making them feel more honest about who they are in general, less like they are living a lie, less burdened by secrecy. If they could stop self-injury altogether, some single women would feel freer to be in an intimate relationship, and those with families would know that loved ones would no longer have to worry. Stopping self-injury would mean that its predecessors — overwhelming emotions, dissociation, flashbacks, nightmares, self-hatred, shame — had been subdued to the point that they could be coped with in healthful ways. Greater emotional stability — a calmness that eludes them — might be theirs. Their current emotional states sometime resemble a roller-coaster ride: up then plummeting down, over and over, in a sickening, taxing cycle. They long to get off and walk on even ground.

Some of the very women who expressed these hopes have now achieved them. One and a half to five years after the original interviews, I was able to recontact nine of the women who had been injuring themselves at the time of the interviews. I often heard heartening tales of improvement and recovery from voices that sounded full and cheerful, contrasting with the sometimes audible shame, anxiety, and distress of the original interviews. Two of my informants have decreased self-injury, five have stopped self-injury altogether, and four of those five have also stopped feeling the need to self-injure.

Esther, now forty-two, has not cut herself for two years. The cutting and the urge seem to have fallen away, she says, although she sometimes "thinks about it," remembering that it was a release. Esther's recovery coincided with giving up one of her two jobs and came after much prayer for relief. She attributes her recovery to prayer and faith, and remembers that she used to look at her arms and think, "God loves me even though I do this to myself." Esther is now a representative of a cosmetics company and enjoys showing other women ways to care for their skin and "helping them feel good about themselves" — so different from her sense of self in her days of self-injury.

Karen, now fifty-two, stopped cutting herself around age forty-eight, a time when she was starting to go back to school to get her master's degree in social work. Karen feels that her therapy supported a view that she was ill, whereas school drew on positive inner resources Karen knew she had but had not been able to tap. Also, learning about other people's patterns of problems helped her understand her own. Karen no longer feels an urge to cut herself and is on no medication. Now a therapist herself, she tries to treat her clients as she would like to have been treated.

Erica, now age forty-six, stopped cutting and hitting herself when she was forty-five. Like Esther, Erica "thinks about it" but does not do it. The turning point came when she tried group therapy for self-injury, something she had long sought as a possibly healing resource. To her surprise, she felt that the group's therapy approach was not going to help her and she stopped attending. She then realized that she had tried every outside help available in her area and had only one resource left: herself. Feeling that this was her last chance, Erica stopped hoping for or relying on outside support. She put all her efforts into thinking about actual safe and comforting situations in her daily life rather than letting herself hit or cut, and succeeded in overcoming her need to self-injure.

Peggy, now thirty-seven, had not banged her head or otherwise injured herself for four months at the time of our last correspondence, when she wrote to me the following:

. . . .

In answer to your question about how I am, I am doing great. I actually have been dealing with another very difficult situation. I got engaged and bought a house, but things went bad and I now have a restraining order. I am concerned about being able to remain in the house. But what is different is that I am not overwhelmed by these feelings. I have a wonderful support system which I have learned to call on when needed. I do not feel isolated and alone. Since I made the move to get out of the relationship, my self-injury has stopped. It has been about four months. What is even better is that whenever I have thoughts of hurting myself I think, "No, I like myself too much to hurt myself." Increased self esteem and better ability in dealing with emotion seems to be the key for me.

. . . .

Elizabeth, now twenty-eight, first stopping cutting and hitting herself when she was twenty-six. Her story of recovery is unique among my informants because our interviews were divided into before and after her recovery, with a year and a half in between. When I first met her, Elizabeth was immersed in self-injury. The only other release she could think of was to "cease existing," which she tried several times to do. In fact, our earlier series of interviews were interrupted because Elizabeth again attempted suicide and was hospitalized. Yet, eighteen months later, she had stopped all cutting and hitting, and was eating regular meals rather than starving, binge-eating, and purging. She was able to tell me the following story by letter and in person.

Six months of a spiral into despair and suicide preceded Elizabeth's recovery. Shortly after being released from a five-week stay at a psychiatric hospital, she cut herself badly, called her psychiatrist, and continued to hack at herself in spite of her therapist's efforts by phone to make her drop the blade. She was rehospitalized and, upon release, was left without a roof over her head because her roommate and friends could no longer tolerate her self-injury. Elizabeth turned to a respite program, which she liked but where she felt tortured because she was trapped inside her body with no release through self-cutting. Every night she thought of hanging herself by her sheets, but checks every five minutes by the night custodian thwarted her. From the respite program she was sent to a less structured house from which she fled after one night, armed with prescribed pills that she planned to take if her future plans did not work out. Elizabeth then moved in with her former fiance but, after confiding in one of her former nurses about her plans with the prescribed pills, was sent back to the respite program, and from there to the psychiatric hospital she hated. While at the hospital, she frantically searched for something to cut herself with but could find nothing sharp enough. She eventually used her own fingernails and spent most of her time there in restraints.

When Elizabeth was released to the respite program again, she was determined to give it her all. She got to know the residents and staff well, and became friends with her roommate there. The staff began to see a big change in her. Just as improvement seemed to be going smoothly, Elizabeth was told that her insurance had run out and that an ambulance was waiting to take her to a mental health center. She was devastated and the staff regretful, yet there was no choice but for her to go. Nonetheless, Elizabeth did relatively well, and in two weeks she was free. She lived with a friend temporarily and drove every day to a day-treatment program where a coordinator helped her through severe flashbacks. Elizabeth then moved to a cozy house that she shared with two other women and returned to work part-time while continuing the day-program.

Elizabeth could feel herself getting stronger, but simultaneously she felt something gnawing at her. She had stopped cutting herself but felt much more suicidal. She fought those feelings, but every night as she went to sleep she prayed that she would not awaken. A blackness came over her life, and she became obsessed with the idea of dying. Then her best friend and her therapist happened to leave town during the same week. Elizabeth swallowed two half-bottles of over-the-counter pills and was hospitalized, but then, to her therapist's dismay, was allowed to leave the hospital after only one night. The following night, after a futile attempt to sleep, Elizabeth jumped out of bed, put seven full bottles of pills into her car, drove to a harbor, and swallowed all but one bottle. Two hours later, the police found her. She stopped breathing in the ambulance and was resuscitated, but in the hospital she slipped into a coma from which doctors expected her not to awaken or to awaken with irreparable brain damage or kidney failure. Elizabeth did awaken, only to find that the 24-hour sitter at her bedside had fallen asleep and that all her belongings, including the last bottle of pills, were on the floor next to her bed. Elizabeth grabbed the pills, swallowed them, and fell into another coma. She awakened again after two days, amazingly suffering no lasting internal damage of any kind. The doctor contacted Elizabeth's parents at their home across the Atlantic and told them that they should come and take Elizabeth home. Five weeks later her brother, who was living in the United States, drove Elizabeth directly from the hospital to the airport and flew with her to their parents' home.

Elizabeth's recovery may have begun during the two comas. For those entire four days her brother, who had raped her when she was fifteen, was at her side, holding her hand, talking to her, crying. Her nurse later told her about her brother's constant presence. Part of Elizabeth's brain may have heard her brother. When she awakened from her second coma, she saw at her bedside her brother, friends, and therapists — sad, worried, angry, and upset, thinking that she was going to die. Elizabeth had believed that no one cared whether she was alive or dead. She learned otherwise.

Once home with her family, Elizabeth could not keep her cutting a secret. When she cut her leg, her sisters knew about it and were disgusted, angry, and did not want to be around her. Elizabeth hates to have people angry with her. She contrasts her family's anger to the response she received during the prior months in the United States. She says that during those months, when she needed help she did not know how to ask for it in words. She knew that if she cut herself, her psychiatrist, therapist, and day-program coordinator would immediately respond with aid. When her family responded with anger, Elizabeth began to think, "Well, what's the point in doing it if it's not going to get me any satisfaction?" She decided to wait and injure herself when she could hide it from her family.

During this waiting period, Elizabeth stayed in the house of her childhood abuse, sleeping in the very bed in which her brother had raped her, bravely re-exposing herself to feared scenes and situations. Elizabeth also took other steps that were possibly part of her healing, though she may not have realized it at the time. First, she became a part of her sisters' and mother's domestic routines. Her mother and sisters paid no attention to what went on inside Elizabeth because they were not in the habit of talking about emotions. Baking, cooking, and cleaning were the important things in life, and Elizabeth let baking, cooking, and cleaning become important to her.

Second, Elizabeth violated the secrecy of self-injury. Because she did not want to go around her parents' house having to constantly hide her scars, she said to her mother, "I want to show you these so that I can take my sweater off and not be afraid of your reaction." Her mother looked at the scars and was horrified, and her horror upset Elizabeth. When her mother saw that Elizabeth was getting upset she said, "They're not *too* bad; they're ugly to look at but not revolting." So, her family got used to the scars, seeing them as part of Elizabeth. Her nephews and nieces saw them, too, and were told that Elizabeth had been in an accident.

Third, Elizabeth shared her struggle with someone. While in her parents' home she craved cutting and asked her mother to go to the bathroom and take all the razors out. Her mother complied and was not angry but grateful that Elizabeth had turned to her. Her gratitude supported Elizabeth's effort. Elizabeth, having taken responsibility for herself by asking for help verbally and by sharing her dilemma with someone, was encouraged by her own actions, so different from the silent, secret cutting of the past. Letting someone else see that she was trying to stop gave her an ally.

Fourth, Elizabeth confronted her father, who used to "mess with" the five-year-old Elizabeth and her sister while the girls were having their baths. In addition, he repeatedly punched and kicked them during drunken rages. During Elizabeth's return home, her father came home drunk a few times and brought up the past, saying, "I don't know why you do that. You're such a beautiful girl. Why do you want to throw your life away like that?" Elizabeth got angry and responded, "Don't you know anything? It's because of *you*; it's because of what you did and the way you treated me. I had no self-worth." He would keep saying, "No, no, you're wrong, you're wrong. You were a perfect daughter before you left [for America], and when you came home you were different." Elizabeth thinks that nonetheless, deep inside, her father knows the truth.

Fifth, Elizabeth's anger toward her brother subsided. Her brother had raped her and since then called her by the name "Ugly." Upon seeing Elizabeth in a coma, he changed. At their home after Elizabeth's suicide attempt, they talked about the event and he said, "I'll never forget as long as I live seeing you lie on that bed." He connects somewhat Elizabeth's suffering with what he did to her. He brought the subject up a few times but tried to justify the rape by saying it was innocent curiosity. Elizabeth thinks that that is his way of apologizing. He also admitted to feeling guilty, and he and Elizabeth are now on better terms. Elizabeth, who used to want to see him suffer, now feels no anger or resentment toward him. She does not want him to feel guilty, because she forgives him, saying, "It's over."

Sixth, Elizabeth actively sought outside help. While waiting to be able to cut again, Elizabeth became suicidal because she did not cut to release her emotions. She also hated being back home and sleeping in the room where she had been raped. She wanted to die and, because she was on medication, had the pills that she could have used for suicide. She would think, "God, I want to take them, I want to take them, I want to take them." She did not confide in her family; therefore, no one there helped her hold back. She had to take the initiative: get up, leave the room, seek help. The Samaritans — a group of volunteers trained to offer emotional support — became her resource. Almost every night, she would go into town, sit in the Samaritans' office, and talk with the volunteers for hours. It became a routine; she had to have an outlet, and she had nothing else. The Samaritans simply listened as long as she needed them. They would say, "What do you think you need at this point?" and Elizabeth came up with ideas by herself. She contrasts this with her psychiatrist and therapist in the United States, who did her thinking for her: "You're feeling this and you're feeling that, and you feel suicidal so we're going to put you in the hospital." With the Samaritans, Elizabeth interpreted her feelings herself. During this period of "waiting" for the freedom and privacy to cut herself again, Elizabeth realized that she no longer needed to.

Upon returning to the United States, Elizabeth joined a self-help group for depression called AWARE and was much supported for her efforts to feel better and stay alive. After her return, she also stopped having full-blown flashbacks. Yet sometimes when she lay in bed in quiet darkness, images would start to come into her mind. Instead of allowing them to overwhelm her, she shouted at them. "No! Get out of my head! I don't want you! I don't need you!" Then she would get up, walk around, turn on the television, read, or listen to music—anything to distract her mind. Now, the images do go away, though they did not at first. It took hard work.

Before her recovery, Elizabeth could not express any emotion. She would want to cry, try to force out tears, but could not. Now, she cries "at the drop of a hat." Before her recovery, anger frightened her and she could not express it except by cutting herself. Now, Elizabeth uses words to say why she is angry and, if necessary, can confront someone else. She calls her verbal anger constructive and healthy. She also taught herself to play the piano, and making music remains an important outlet. Before her recovery, Elizabeth thought she was "not good enough" to treat herself well or to undertake things she enjoyed. Now, she takes a hot bubble bath when she wishes, gives herself a manicure or facial, and appreciates her body. When Elizabeth looks at her scars nowadays she thinks, "That was me back then that did all that." Elizabeth once contemplated having plastic surgery on her arm, which sometimes feels disconnected from her body because of the forearm's deep cuts and muscle damage. Doctors have told her that the grooves are too deep to repair, and Elizabeth has learned to accept her scars.

Yet, at times, old messages try to intervene: "Who do you think you are? You think you're doing so well now. You're not worth that much." Elizabeth used to listen to such thoughts, but she can fight them now. Instead of trusting such internal messages she asks other people, "Do you think I am ugly?" or "Do you think I'm a bad person?" Always the responses make her feel better. When she is alone and looks in the mirror, she still cannot stand what she sees. But she now tries hard to find something she likes about her body, and she walks away from the mirror thinking about that one good thing; she does not walk away wanting to cut herself.

Elizabeth thinks that her life will continue to change now that she has stopped injuring herself, and that she has much to make up for. She wants to socialize and enjoy other things that she could not enjoy because she was so absorbed in self-injury. She has already begun pursuing a career in psychology so that she can help people who self-injure, not only as a therapist but also as an advocate who can share her experiences and her recovery with others:

. . . .

I know it's part of my past; it's no longer a part of me now — it's gone. But I don't regret it because I had to go through it to learn, and I learned a lot from it. I learned how to take care of myself and it feels good taking care of myself in a good way. Because people respect you more, you respect yourself.

. . . .

The scars and her past are not going to stop Elizabeth from pursuing her career in psychology, but she is somewhat apprehensive. Sometimes she asks herself, "Do I have a right to do psychology when I was so screwed up?" Then she answers her own question: "I'm not screwed up now; I got myself well and on my feet, and now maybe I can help people from my experience." But she sometimes still hears a nagging voice in the back of her head saying, "You're carrying the scars; how can you go be a psychologist when you have scars that were self-inflicted?" But Elizabeth remains undeterred.

While she was going through her own overwhelming difficulties, Elizabeth felt unable to take care of a child. Now that she has learned to take good care of herself, she feels able to take care of others: "I know I would be a good mother now and I want to have children; that's a major thing for me."

Elizabeth left our last interview with both of us happy and amazed at the change in her. As planned, a few days later she moved to a different city and began a new professional life as a client care coordinator at a home health agency. Even though the work was hectic, she loved it. When she went home at night, she thought it ironic that she was now taking care of people when, for so long, she was the one needing care. She kept her past to herself, however, because there was no one in her new environment whom she knew or trusted enough for confidences. Elizabeth also realized that she had never really known her roommate, a friend of four years, and did not enjoy sharing an apartment with her. Dislocation, secrecy, a new job, and loneliness — difficult for the most serene minds — began to take their toll on Elizabeth. At that point, seven months after she had told me the story of her gradual recovery, Elizabeth sent me the following letter:

. . . .

For a while I was doing so well. I was eating healthy meals and not cutting at all. I was even enjoying being healthy. But the lonelier I got the harder it was for me. I started cutting a few nights ago and the pleasure I got from it was intense. Nobody in the entire world knows (except you now). I just don't feel people would understand. They think that once you're in recovery, they don't have to worry about you anymore — you're not allowed to have a bad day, or feel down once in a while. People get scared and they run away. It's too hard for them the second time around. I have about ten mothers in work who bug me about eating and they never back off. My boss told me I definitely do not have a poker face — I can't hide any emotions. She's right, but I wish I could. So every so often I slice into my wonderfully scarred arm and I can paint a smile on my face and they all leave me alone. Secrecy can be a wonderful thing. . . .

I started going to see a psychologist but I stopped because I felt as though if I shared my deepest secrets, she would put me into a hospital. So there was no point in going anymore — secrecy is bad in therapy. I wish I had just one person that had no control over me who would listen without judgement and not try to change me or fix me. I would pour out my darkest secrets with no holds barred and I bet that would feel really good.

I visited my family . . . about a month ago and even though I had a nice time, it made me realize I would never belong there. So then when I returned here and felt like I had no one here, that's when I started to feel like this. I'm so tired of wandering and ending up nowhere. I'm tired of pretending, and this whole world is full of pretence. Don't you think?

I know you have the mind of a psychologist but I don't think of you as that. I think of you as someone who listened without judging and that was nice for me, (even though it was an interview).

I had just started getting used to wearing short sleeves and not being ashamed and now it's 85 degrees outside and I'm covered up again. Nobody can see my fresh cuts — anyway, they're for my pleasure alone. But, I do still have a grasp on reality. I know I'm heading for trouble but for now I don't care about all that. I just care about gaining some control again.

I think a lot about dying and I wish God would take me, but I don't think I can die at my own hands-not now anyway. I would have to break my ties with some people first so they wouldn't get so upset and then I wouldn't feel so guilty. But for now, I'm too close to my family and they would be too upset with me. . . .

Every now and then I drive to . . . [the] beach. It looks out onto the . . . skyline and it's incredibly beautiful. I sit on a rock and look at all that wonder and I think — that's how I feel, on the outside looking in. All I could see were flickering lights and [all I could] hear [was] a car horn and I was so far away from that. Life, everything was going on in the city and here I was on my rock, watching from the outside. That's how it is with me and the world. And no matter what I do, I just cannot fit in. So I will probably give up trying and just be a freak on the outside with bloody marks up and down her arms.

God, it feels so good to put all this on paper and get it out of my head!

But I will end now and hope you will write to me soon. . . .

        . . . .

I responded to Elizabeth's letter, then later on sent her a card, and six months after the letter quoted above she wrote me again. She had decided, she said, that she could not afford to use self-injury again, calling it a "road to destruction." She fought against her impulses, "took things very, very slowly," and was able, once again, to stop injuring herself. Feeling that the living situation with her roommate was jeopardizing her mental health, she moved out and took an apartment with a very compatible colleague. Elizabeth also wrote that she has been through discovery of a large tumor (benign), surgery, and severe pain, and finds resisting self-injury a daily battle. She has had 24-hour postoperative care at home from the nurses she works with, care that has bonded all involved. She feels that this time around, in spite of the enormous stresses of physical disability and pain, she is winning the battle against self-injury. Two letters written three and seven months later, and her critique of this chapter a year later, confirm this.

Elizabeth's first recovery taught her useful lessons. She emerged from a death-like unconsciousness to find loving concern on all faces, not the indifference she expected. Knowing that others care about her influences her current thoughts and behavior: now, when she is suicidal, she restrains herself because she feels the ties to her family and refuses to put them through such pain again. Elizabeth also learned to use words to ask for help. Fortunately, she found the Samaritans and a self-help group, two resources that encouraged self-sufficiency, exerted no control, and were always available. During her relapse, she suspected that a therapist would not offer the same quality of nonthreatening succor, chose not to confide in a therapist, then gave up the idea of therapy altogether. Elizabeth felt that honest words would not have been safe, leaving her speechless once more. Fortunately, she was strong enough to recover again from self-injury, perhaps remembering the self-sufficiency she had acquired during her first recovery.

Elizabeth's relapse was not surprising considering her experience of three simultaneous major stresses: a new city, a new job and profession, and an incompatible roommate. Like other signs of emotional distress such as depression and obsessive-compulsive disorder, self-injury can recur when a woman faces new stresses, requiring further self-help or competent, experienced, nonthreatening outside help to overcome it again. During her recovery from disability and pain, Elizabeth managed to remain free of self-injury. Possibly, the important move away from an incompatible roommate to a compatible one and the loving concern and care offered by her colleagues helped her through.

Elizabeth's story has no ending. After her surgery, she had to fight recurring strong urges to injure herself. She succeeded in spite of major surgery, disability, and pain, and says that these experiences have made her stronger. Life may put further severe stresses in Elizabeth's path, and years from now she may again find it difficult or impossible to avoid self-injury. Possibly, for some women, freedom from self-injury requires a lifetime of vigilance: recognizing triggering stresses and reminding oneself how to overcome them. Also, the constant, brief, repeated, and almost unconscious self-injury of picking, chewing, pinching, and quick hitting may require different recovery methods from the more intermittent episodes of cutting, burning, and severe or sustained hitting. Elizabeth is one of increasing numbers of women who are documenting their recovery so that their experiences can help others.

Elizabeth's recovery has points in common with Meredith's, Helena's, and Sarah O.'s stories (chapters 3, 6, and 8), and with Karen's, Peggy's, and Erica's experiences — points worth highlighting because of their possible usefulness for self-injuring women and their therapists:

1. Feeling a connection to others was cited as one reason for stopping and remaining free of self-injury and for staying alive. Elizabeth stopped cutting herself partly to avert her family's anger, and later said that she could not kill herself because her death would be too upsetting to her family and close friends. Of her serious suicide attempt she now says, "I didn't want to put anyone through that again." This was a new perception to Elizabeth, who had thought her death would hardly matter. Similarly, Sarah O. says that one reason she does not want to cut herself is that it upsets the people around her: "There are consequences to my cutting; it doesn't just affect me. . . ." In particular, Sarah O. values her long-term partner who has made it clear that there is not room in their partnership for cutting. Meredith, too, has discovered that mutual care and trust between therapist and client can keep her from self-injury: "Her trust in me and her trust that I will keep my word and my relationship with her is more important to me and does more for me than my cutting does. I never thought that there would be something that would be able to replace that."

2. Specific future goals in life deemed incompatible with self-injury supported the determination to stop. Meredith, who stands at the beginning of a

career in social work, reminds herself that she wants to be in recovery in order to help others. Helena and Elizabeth say that they want to have families and be free of self-injury when they do.

3. Life events taught empowerment and increased self-esteem. Karen went back to school, Peggy ended a destructive relationship, and Erica turned to her own inner resources. All three circumstances showed these women that they are not helpless and dependent, that they are competent and can defend themselves — the opposite of their childhood helplessness.

4. Conventional and unconventional talk therapy helped some of them express past experiences and present emotions in words, integrate past and present, understand why they self-injure, learn positive thought patterns and self-reliance, and discover that someone could care about them without also hurting them.

5. Alternative coping strategies were learned and practiced.

Stopping self-injury is a major step forward and has improved the self-esteem and quality of life of those women — Elizabeth, Helena, Esther, Karen, Erica, and Sarah O. — who have experienced recovery over time. Those who have stopped but still feel the urge to self-injure want to also overcome that urge so that they will not have to expend their energy resisting. When the urge itself subsides, a woman can be permanently free of self-injury, or a major stress later in life can rekindle the urge or cause a relapse. But strengths and strategies to stop self-injury, once learned, can be remobilized: self-injury can recur and be overcome again.

Epilogue

Three Faces of Self-Injury

As THE preceding chapters illustrate, repeatedly cutting, hitting, or otherwise injuring the body is now generally viewed through the lens of psychology and seen as socially unacceptable. However, psychology is only one context for discussing self-injury. People past and present have given deliberate self-injury different names depending on the circumstances and on the prevailing attitudes of the time.

Fashion is a term now used for some self-injuries. Piercing, scarring, and tattooing the skin are part of a growing practice sometimes called "body art" or "body modification." Ritually or privately performed for centuries in some cultures, these practices have gained recent popularity in parts of the Western world. Tattoos or scars as body adornments and jewelry for piercings are now common sights. The pain involved is considered a necessary evil like the pain of other fashions past and present: plucking eyebrows, injecting collagen, undergoing cosmetic surgery, or wearing corsets, narrow shoes, and high heels.

A simple wish to adorn the body can call for rings hanging from various parts of the face or torso. As part of that fashion, a person may add a new piercing and ring to mark a certain time span or event, such as the birth of a child. However, the wish to cause pain or feel it can also enter into the wish to pierce or cut others or to be pierced or cut. In this context, piercing and cutting are also called *blood sports*. Being pierced or cut can lead to high physical excitement or to an altered state experienced as pleasurable and sometimes spiritual. When this occurs, the event seems to cross boundaries between a fashion statement and a compulsion or addiction. The event can be addictive because of the sensations it produces, and yet become a fashion statement if a ring goes through the piercing or if tattoo ink is rubbed into an artistic design cut into the skin. Some professional piercers notice that many of their female clients interpret nipple- or labia-piercing as a ritual to reclaim their bodies after experiencing sexual trauma.[1] Some body artists who publicly perform cuttings and piercings remark that people who cannot express something in words express themselves with other symbols,[2] bringing such performances within the realm of psychology. Yet, body artists often do not use negative prior experiences to explain why a person would choose to be cut or pierced by a professional or engage in sadomasochism. Important, instead, is simply the discovery that pain can become pleasure, which in turn can become a spiritual experience. Some body artists think that tattooing, piercing, cutting, and other body modifications reveal possibilities in the brain and body that have been neglected in Western cultures.[3] They want to explore such possibilities.

Some people who have their skin pierced, scarred, or tattooed find that they want that experience again and again. The event, not the result, is central. Voluntarily subjugating the body to the intense sensation of pain or life-threatening distress can lead to a separation of thoughts and feelings from the body. The mind can go into a trance or even separate itself and observe the body, feeling no pain. The trance or out-of-body state can be euphoric and, perhaps, addictive.

An American advertising executive who has taken the name Fakir Musafar discovered this euphoria during his boyhood. As a child, Musafar often went into what he describes as spontaneous trance states and wanted to feel strong sensations in his body. When he was six a carnival came to his town, and Musafar saw a man being tattooed. Instantly, he wanted to mark and pierce his body, to feel "odd sensations."[4] After years of secretly subjecting his body to piercings, tattooing, constrictions, stretchings, and weights, Musafar has become well-known for photographs, videos, and performances of his "body play." Musafar's practices are sometimes copied from those of cultures within New Guinea and India where some people demonstrate altered states by flinging themselves onto beds of thorns and rolling in them, lying on sharp blades, hanging by flesh hooks, and sewing small weights onto the skin. He has also studied former American Indian rituals in which the object was to use physical ordeals to achieve other-worldly experiences such as visions.

Fakir Musafar enjoys the dissociation of mind and body and considers himself trained in dissociation. At times, his senses have floated upward and looked down as his body bore numerous spears, or looked back at his body lashed to a wall: "The part of me that thinks, and feels, and sees, and hears, and answers to a name was at least ten feet from that wall! What was I looking at? Was it me? Or was I the 'looker'?"[5] He calls some out-of-body states "having an ecstasy."[6] If he cannot feel the transition to an altered state just before a performance, he will not perform.

Rather than trying a variety of body modifications, some people use only tattooing. This practice sometimes begins with having one tattoo, then repeatedly coming back for more, eventually tattooing the entire body—including genitals and face. Tattoos can signify belonging to a group, such as a group of seamen, or signify alienation, when tattoos are used as visual proof of being outside society. At times, tattoos are associated with a love of the rite-of-passage aspect of the tattooing process; with the ability to bear pain; or with spontaneous out-of-body states, sometimes interpreted as religious events because they mirror some saints' experiences.

Deliberate self-injury can, indeed, be seen through the lens of religion: it is still a regular practice in some religious settings. Self-inflicted renouncement, abnegation, suffering, and detachment are found in Buddhism, Islam, Judaism, and Christianity.[7] Within the Catholic church, self-injury is called *body mortification*. Mortifications are meant to control or punish bodily passions and appetites through abstinence, discomfort, or self-inflicted pain. They can include denial of the sensuous pleasures of looking at views; smelling flowers; eating tasty food; sleeping in clean, comfortable beds; masturbating; or making love. One step beyond denials are discomforts or abstinences such as sleeping in a rigid position, vigils, or fasting. The most severe mortification is to deliberately self-inflict pain. Methods range from kneeling with bare knees erect on the floor in prayer, to self-flagellation. One former nun described what is called "the discipline": self-flagellation on the buttocks and legs three times weekly with either a lighter whip meant to hurt but leave no traces, or a heavier one that can draw blood.[8]

In the Middle Ages, self-inflicted discomfort or pain was considered an appropriate act toward the body and toward God. Besides foregoing food and sleep, monks would wear hair shirts, chain mail, and metal plates; whip themselves; and roll in thorn bushes and nettles. These ascetic practices were meant to subdue sexual desires, expiate guilt, express devotion, and avoid punishment after death. Some monks considered asceticism a training for paradise: learning to achieve indifference to physical needs and suffering, to be above or outside the body, and therefore in perfect peace.[9] Eventually, many of these practices spread to the general population, some of whom went on pilgrimages barefoot or on their knees, in sackcloth, and carrying metal weights or a wooden cross.[10] Some people inflicted wounds on themselves to imitate the stigmata of Christ.

One eleventh-century ascetic was renowned because of his body mortifications. His very name, Dominic Loricatus, is derived from the *lorica*, heavy metal plates that he increased over time to eight hanging on his neck, hips, and legs.[11] He turned the reciting of the Psalters into a ritual of self-injury: for every ten Psalms he would whip himself a thousand times, and for every fifteen perform one hundred genuflexions.[12] Loricatus regularly recited the Psalters twenty times every six days. He is said to have carried the wounds of Christ on his body.

Accounts of self-injury within religious settings continued after the Middle Ages. Two especially well-documented accounts concern sixteenth and seventeenth-century Italian women. Orsola Giuliani, born in 1660, was influenced by her mother's piety and by accounts of the saints' lives. Around age three, feeling a desire to suffer, she put her hand in a firepot so that it would burn like the martyred saints. Having heard of a saint who, as a child, punished herself by closing a trunk on her finger, Orsola "played around" by putting her hand in the open front door until the door was accidentally shut on her fingers. "But these things were mere notions, without any understanding," she later said.[13] She apparently was prone to cuts and bruises and would secretly walk on her knees, lick the ground to make crosses, stand with outstretched arms for long periods, and flagellate herself with apron strings tied in knots. In describing the secret nature of these acts, she said, "I wanted no one to see me. . . . I did all sorts of things, but without the light of God, because I did not understand what I was doing. I only watched that no one would know."[14]

The idea of marrying revolted Orsola, who wanted only to enter a convent and did so at age seventeen, becoming Sister Veronica. At the convent, Veronica bore a heavy wooden yoke on her shoulders and a large rock on her tongue, and beat herself with chains and sharply-studded flagellating instruments. She also reports that a devil took her form and went around saying bad things, making Veronica's superior angry.[15] Only with difficulty could Veronica convince her superior that evil apparitions were about. She wrote that demons would slap her, knock her off ladders, and bite and kick her. In her mid-thirties, wounds appeared on Sister Veronica's hands, feet, and breasts. Until it became clear that the wounds would not stop bleeding, her confessors were suspicious that the wounds were self-inflicted rather than a sign from God. Although Sister Veronica was eventually canonized, during her lifetime the church could not decide whether she was a saint or a witch.

As a child, Mary Magdalen de'Pazzi, a devout, sixteenth-century Florentine, would fast; wear a crown of thorns; whip herself; and, before going to bed, tie a prickly belt around her body. When she was ten, she made a vow of virginity and chastity and, after puberty, entered a convent where she burned herself with hot wax and continued to whip herself, sometimes with a chain. While a nun, she would periodically writhe and convulse on the floor while experiencing hallucinations of being attacked and beaten. She suffered from involuntary lascivious thoughts and lewd images that drove her to roll naked in thorns or whip herself until she bled. She would also ask other nuns to whip, slap, spank, and walk upon her. Sixty-two years after her death she was canonized.[16]

"Saint" is not a designation a self-injuring woman receives today. A woman who repeatedly injures herself often finds that others view her actions through the lens of psychology and psychiatry, not through the lens of fashion, religion, or a search for the spirituality of trance or out-of-body states. Yet, religious and psychiatric self-injury have striking similarities: both can involve shifting levels of consciousness; hearing, seeing, feeling, or tasting things that others do not; and altered perceptions of one's own body, one's surroundings, and time. In both cases, self-injury can be a release of mounting tension, either voluntary tension achieved through ritual music, chanting, or dance, or the involuntary tensions produced by life events. In both cases, self-injury is often not perceived as painful because the mind is already in a trance-like state.

In ritual contexts, a person often willingly injures or allows her- or himself to be injured in the belief that the injuries are beneficial to the person or the community. The Christian religion is based on such a belief, as were many pagan religions before it. Similarly, some people who undergo private or public body modifications seem to believe that being extensively tattooed or doing unusual things to the body are necessary to keep them from becoming socially dangerous. Anton LaVey, who founded the Church of Satan where rituals are performed, says that body modifications are "a safety valve, a way of keeping yourself—not on the straight and narrow, certainly, but from maybe being a mass murderer!"[17] Some people who are considered mentally ill in Western cultures say that they injure themselves because it is, at least temporarily, beneficial to themselves, and perhaps to their communities.[18] Similarly, several of my informants say that they injure themselves not only because it brings release to them, but because they are afraid that they might otherwise harm others. Self-injury enables them to remain members of society rather than dangers to society. Pope Pius XII could have been speaking for self-injuring women rather than for Catholic doctrine when he said that a person can "allow parts to be destroyed or mutilated . . . to ensure his being's existence and to avoid or . . . to repair serious and lasting damage which cannot otherwise be avoided or repaired."[19]

Self-injury in all three contexts—as fashionable/spiritual body art, religious body mortification, and psychiatric phenomenon—can avert chaos and establish order, at least temporarily. In some social and cultural settings, self-injury is accepted and even welcomed as a way of protecting society and expiating sins. One of the challenges for self-injuring women's families, friends, and caregivers is to understand that abuse-related self-injury serves a personal and social need for temporarily re-establishing order, but is also an emotionally painful problem and a sign of unspoken distress. Such understanding might alleviate self-injury's effects on women's partnerships, family lives, and friendships and relieve self-injuring women from the burdens of secrecy and social ostracism.

Resources

In the United States, Canada, and England

Groups and Programs

Boston Women's Health Book Collective
240 Elm Street
Somerville, MA 02144 USA
Telephone: (617) 625-0277 (for appointments)

Library containing books and articles on self-injury and related topics is open, by appointment, to the public.

Bristol Crisis Service for Women
P.O. Box 654
Bristol, BS99 1XH UK
Telephone: 0117 925 1119 (from the United States dial 011-44-117-925-1119)
Web site: http://www.users.zetnet.co.uk/bcsw/

Booklets, information sheets, and a help-line on Fridays and Saturdays from 9:00 P.M. to 12:30 A.M. GMT.

Independent Living Center of the North Shore and Cape Ann, Inc.
27 Congress St., Suite 107
Salem, MA 01970 USA
Telephone: (888) 751-0077 (voice and TTY)
(978) 741-0077 (voice and TTY)
Fax: (978) 741-1133
Email: ilcnsc@rkaol.com

Offers education, advocacy, and support on issues related to self-injury for people who self-injure and their family members, friends, and therapists; publisher of the *Women and Self-Injury Resource Guide*.

EMDR (Eye Movement Desensitization and Reprocessing) Institute, Inc.
P.O. Box 51010
Pacific Grove, CA 93950 USA
Telephone: (831) 372-3900
Fax: (408) 647-9881
Email: inst@emdr.com
Web site: http://www.emdr.com

Provides information on EMDR and names of therapists in various areas of the United States who offer EMDR.

National Self-Harm Network
P.O. Box 16190
London, NW 13WW UK
Telephone: 0171-916-5472 (from the United States dial 011-44-171-916-5472)

Part of a group called Survivors Speak Out, 34 Osnaburgh Street, London NW1 3ND. Campaigns for rights and keeps record of poor treatment of people who self-injure. Offers self-help sheet and lists of resources throughout the United Kingdom. This group and the Bristol Crisis Service for Women can give information about many other groups in the United Kingdom and also have some information about resources in Europe.

S.A.F.E. (Self-Abuse Finally Ends) Alternatives
7115 W. North Ave., Suite 319
Oak Park, IL 60302 USA
Telephone: 1-800-DONTCUT or 1-888-306-SAFE

You can request a return call and a packet of information about self-injury and about the S.A.F.E. thirty-day treatment program.

S.A.F.E. (Self-Abuse Finally Ends) in Canada
Mary Graham, executive director
306-241 Simcoe Street
London, Ontario
Canada N6B 3L4
Telephone: (519) 434-9473

Offers a ten-week therapy program for people who injure themselves.

Sidran Foundation
2328 W. Joppa Road, Suite 15
Lutherville, MD 21093 USA
Telephone: (410) 825-8888
Fax: (410) 337-0747
Email: sidran@access.digex.net
Web site: http://www.sidran.org

Provides educational resources on trauma and trauma therapy.

University of Washington Department of Psychology
Behavioral Research and Therapy Clinics
P.O. Box 351525

Seattle, WA 98195-1525 USA
Telephone: (206) 685-2037
Trains therapists to use dialectical behavior therapy (DBT) and provides names of people in various areas of the USA trained in DBT.

Publications
Books

Alderman, Tracy, Ph.D. 1997. *The Scarred Soul: Understanding and Ending Self-Inflicted Violence*. Oakland, Calif.: New Harbinger Publications.

Babiker, Gloria, and Lois Arnold. 1997. *The Language of Injury: Comprehending Self-Mutilation*. Leicester, U.K.: British Psychological Society.

Conterio, Karen and Wendy Lader, Ph.D. 1998. *Bodily Harm: The Breakthrough Treatment Program for Self-Injurers*. New York: Hyperion.

Harrison, Diane. 1996. *Vicious Circles*. London, U.K.: Good Practices in Mental Health.

Levenkron, Steven. 1998. *Cutting: Understanding and Overcoming Self-Mutilation*. New York: W. W. Norton and Company.

Miller, Dusty. 1994. *Women Who Hurt Themselves: A Book of Hope and Understanding*. New York: Basic Books.

Pembroke, Louise Roxanne, ed. 1994. *Self Harm: Perspectives from Personal Experience*. Available through Survivors Speak Out, 34 Osnaburgh Street, London NW1 3ND, U.K. Telephone: 0171 916 5472 (from the United States dial 011-44-171-916-5472).

Spendler, Helen. 1996. *Who's Hurting Who?* Manchester U.K.: 42nd Street.

Trautmann, Kristy, and Robin Connors. 1994. *Understanding Self-Injury: A Workbook for Adults*. Available through Pittsburgh Action Against Rape, 81 South 19th Street, Pittsburgh, PA 15203.

Newsletters

The Cutting Edge
P.O. Box 20819
Cleveland, Ohio 44120

Raising Issue
Although this newsletter is no longer in print, you can obtain from a back issue "Assessment of Self-Injurious Coping Behaviors" by David K. Sakheim and Lorraine J. Stanek. The material in this article is designed to help generate ideas, concepts, and insights about self-injury and possible alternatives. Send a self-addressed, stamped, business-sized envelope with your request to:

David K. Sakheim, Ph.D.
1610 Ellington Road
South Windsor, CT (USA) 06074-2701

SASH (Survivors of Self-Abuse and Self-Harming)
20 Lackmore Road
Enfield
Middlesex, EN1 4PB UK

SHOUT (Self-Harm Overcome by Understanding and Tolerance)
Bristol Crisis Service for Women
P.O. Box 654
Bristol BS99 1XH UK
Telephone: 0117 925 1119 (from the United States dial 011-44-117-925-1119)

Audio and Video Tapes

Understanding and Treating the Self-Injurious Patient: A Guide to Assessment and Intervention Strategies. 1997. Developed by the Self Abuse Finally Ends (S.A.F.E.) Alternatives Program. Call 1-800-DONTCUT to request an order form for the audiotape.

Between the Lines: A Documentary About Cutting. 1997. Videotape by Sophie Constantinou. Available through:
Sophie Constantinou
131 Albion St., #6
San Francisco, CA 94110 USA
Telephone: (415) 431-7203
Email: sophc@sirius.com

Stigmata: The Transfigured Body. 1991. Videotape by Leslie Asako Gladsjo. 27 minutes. Described in catalogue as a "look at women who are engaged in unusual forms of body modification such as tattooing, cutting, piercing, and branding." Available through:
Women Make Movies, Inc.
462 Broadway, Suite 500
New York, NY 10013 USA
Telephone: (212) 925-0606
Fax: (212) 925-2052

Skin and Ink: Women and Tattooing. 1990. Videotape by Barbara Attie. 28

minutes. Described in catalogue as a "documentary on women who have tattoos and the women who create them. . . . Artists, secretaries, academics, and mothers reveal their motivations to become heavily tattooed, and the social repercussions. . . ." Also available through Women Make Movies, Inc., as listed above.

Resources through Writing

http://www.betterhealth.com

This web site offers weekly support groups on self-injury. One meets on Mondays at 10 P.M. EST (9 P.M. CST, 7 P.M. PST, 3 A.M. GMT). Another, set up to accommodate non-U.S. schedules, meets Wednesdays at 3 P.M. EST (2 P.M. CST, 12 P.M. PST, 8 P.M. GMT).

http://palace.net/-llama/selfinjury

A comprehensive source of self-injury information.
Email: llama@palace.net

The Samaritans

Trained volunteer participants in this nonreligious charity offer emotional support by phone, visit, and letter to the despairing and suicidal. Callers are guaranteed confidentiality and the right to make their own decisions. The Samaritans are now available by email, run through Cheltenham, England.
Email: jo@samaritans.org
Anonymous email: samaritans@anon.twwells.com

SASH (Survivors of Abuse and Self Harming)

SASH is a pen-friend network for support and friendship on a one-to-one basis.
20 Lackmore Road
Enfield
Middlesex, EN1 4PB UK

An internet search will take you to other sources. Possible topics to look under include self-injury, self-mutilation, self-inflicted violence, self-abuse, and trauma.

Notes

Introduction

1. See Annie G. Rogers, "Writing on their Bodies I: Understanding Self Mutilation with Adolescent Girls through Creative Writing in Psychotherapy," unpublished paper presented at the Harvard Medical School Conference: "Child and Adolescent Self-Destruction," Boston, Mass., February 3, 1996, and at Trinity College: Psychology and Women's Studies Departments, Dublin, Ireland, April 25, 1996.

2. Of the 362 participants in the McLean Study of Adult Development in Belmont, Massachusetts, there were only 16 African Americans, 7 Hispanic Americans, 5 Asian Americans, and 10 of biracial origin, yet proportionally the same percentage of each ethnic group injured themselves as did the Caucasian American participants of European descent. Personal communication, Michelle Haynes, research assistant, 1997.

3. Clinicians have generally seen more female than male self-injuring clients, although one study finds men and women equally likely to self-injure. See John Briere and Eliana Gil, "Self-Mutilation in Clinical and General Population Samples: Prevalence, Correlates, and Functions: in *American Journal of Orthopsychiatry* 68, no. 4 (October 1998), 617. Data gathered from psychiatric clinics and hospitals do not reflect the numbers of incarcerated men who injure themselves.

4. See, for example, Barent W. Walsh and Paul M. Rosen, *Self-Mutilation: Theory, Research, and Treatment* (New York: The Guilford Press, 1988), 10; and Armando R. Favazza, "Why Patients Mutilate Themselves" in *Hospital and Community Psychiatry* 40, no. 2 (1989), 137. The Walsh and Rosen definition includes the statement that self-mutilation is "performed while in a state of psychic crisis," a restriction that I have not found uniformly true. See some of my informants' experiences with self-picking and -hitting, described in chapter one.

5. See John Bayley, "Anything that Burns," an essay in the *London Review of Books* (July 3, 1997), 20, on the Russian writer Venedikt Yerofeev, who died of throat cancer as a result of drinking such concoctions.

6. The *Diagnostic and Statistical Manual of Mental Disorders*, 4th ed., (Washington, D.C.: American Psychiatric Press, 1993), 425, states that "self-destructive and impulsive behavior" and other problems are more commonly associated with interpersonal stressors such as childhood abuse (as opposed to impersonal experiences such as earthquake, fire, etc.). Some researchers consider that a new category called Complex PTSD or Disorder of Extreme Stress Not Otherwise Specified is needed to accurately encompass the manifold symptoms of distress resulting from interpersonal trauma. See Judith Lewis Herman, "Sequelae of Prolonged and Repeated Trauma: Evidence for a Complex Posttraumatic Syndrome (DESNOS)" in Jonathan R. T. Davidson and

Edna B. Foa (eds.), *Posttraumatic Stress Disorder: DSM-IV and Beyond* (Washington, D.C.: American Psychiatric Press, 1993), 213–228.

7. One woman who participated in this project compulsively washes, a second compulsively cleans, and a third occasionally compulsively counts. See also Jose A. Yaryura-Tobias et al., "Self-Mutilation, Anorexia, and Dysmenorrhia in Obsessive Compulsive Disorder," *International Journal of Eating Disorders* 17, no. 1, (1995), 33–38. In some people, skin-picking may be a sign of obsessive-compulsive disorder rather than of self-injury. This is suggested in Dan J. Stein et al., "Compulsive Picking and Obsessive-Compulsive Disorder," *Psychosomatics* 34, no. 2 (1993), 177–181. It is also often associated with hair-pulling (trichotillomania).

8. In 1995, the most recent year for abuse statistics, 2.96 million cases were reported and 1.11 million cases were confirmed. See "Child Maltreatment, 1995," a report on data from the U.S. Department of Health and Human Services National Center of Child Abuse and Neglect, in Michael Petit and Patrick Curtis, *Child Abuse and Neglect: A look at the States. 1997 CWLA Stat Book* (Washington, D.C.: Child Welfare League of America, 1997), 5.

Prologue

1. See John Briere and Marsha Runtz, "The Long-Term Effects of Sexual Abuse: A Review and Synthesis," *New Directions for Mental Health Services* 51 (Fall 1991), 3–13; Beth S. Brodsky et al., "Relationship of Dissociation to Self-Mutilation and Childhood Abuse in Borderline Personality Disorder," *American Journal of Psychiatry* 152, no. 12 (December 1995), 1788–1792; Armando R. Favazza, *Bodies Under Siege: Self-Mutilation in Culture and Psychiatry* (Baltimore: The Johns Hopkins University Press, 1987); Gail S. Greenspan and Seven E. Samuel, "Self-Cutting After Rape," *American Journal of Psychiatry* 146 (June 1989), 789–790; Judith Lewis Herman et al., "Childhood Trauma in Borderline Personality Disorder," *American Journal of Psychiatry* 116, no. 4 (April 1989), 490–495; D. R. Langbehn and B. Pfohl, "Clinical Correlates of Self-Mutilation among Psychiatric Inpatients," *Annals of Clinical Psychiatry* 5, no. 1 (March 1993), 45–51; Ellen Leibenluft et al., "The Inner Experience of the Borderline Self-Mutilator," *Journal of Personality Disorders* 1, no. 4 (1987), 317–324; Charles B. Schaffer et al., "Self-Mutilation and the Borderline Personality," *The Journal of Nervous and Mental Disease* 170, no. 8 (1982), 468–473; Kenneth R. Silk et al., "Borderline Personality Disorder Symptoms and Severity of Sexual Abuse," *American Journal of Psychiatry* 152, no. 7 (July 1995), 1059–1064; and Bessel A. van der Kolk et al., "Childhood Origins of Self-Destructive Behavior," *American Journal of Psychiatry* 148, no. 12 (December 1991), 1667.

2. Trauma that occurs outside the home and during adulthood can also lead to self-injury, as can childhood trauma related to major physical disabilities, illnesses, and repeated hospitalizations. However, because much of the abuse leading to self-injury occurs interpersonally and at home, and because all the women I interviewed experienced such abuse, this chapter focuses on the home.

3. See Bessel A. van der Kolk and Jose Saporta, "The Biological Response to Psychic Trauma: Mechanisms and Treatment of Intrusion and Numbing," *Anxiety Research* 4 (1991), 203. I define trauma as one or more inescapable events causing emotions that interfere with the brain's ability to process information verbally and/or to regulate emotions. This definition is adapted from the study by van der Kolk and Saporta, 199–200 and 202.

4. D. Finkelhor, *Sexually Victimized Children* (New York: Free Press, 1979), as cited in Judith Lewis Herman, J. Christopher Perry, and Bessel A. van der Kolk, "Childhood Trauma in Borderline Personality Disorder," *American Journal of Psychiatry* 146, no. 4 (April 1989), 494.

5. James A. Chu and Diana L. Dill, "Dissociative Symptoms in Relation to Childhood Physical and Sexual Abuse," *American Journal of Psychiatry* 147, no. 7 (July 1990), 887. This article cites eleven studies concerning symptoms related to childhood abuse.

6. Bessel A. Van der Kolk et al., "Childhood Origins of Self-Destructive Behavior," 1667.

7. It appears that suicide attempts before age ten are rare, but that children as young as three can think and talk about a wish to die. See Arthur Schwartz and Ruth M. Schwartz, *Depression: Theories and Treatments* (New York, Columbia University Press, 1993), 365.

8. I am using the general term "dissociation" rather than the specific term "depersonalization" to describe consciousness as being detached from one's body.

9. Bessel A. van der Kolk and Rita E. Fisler, "Childhood Abuse and Neglect and Loss of Self-Regulation," *Bulletin of the Menninger Clinic* 58, no. 2 (1994), 148.

10. In Bessel A. van der Kolk et al., "Childhood Origins of Self-Destructive Behavior," 1669, the authors find dissociation directly associated with cutting.

11. This is true for Mary, who has a suicidal child alter identity, as mentioned in chapter seven.

12. Judith Himber, "Blood Rituals: Self-Cutting in Female Psychiatric Inpatients," *Psychotherapy* 31, no. 4 (Winter 1994), 622.

Chapter 1

1. Information from my own research and from Gina E. Rayfield, "Eating Disorders: A Survivor's Tool for Sexual Abuse," American Anorexia/Bulimia Association, Inc., newsletter, n.d., 6; and Craig Johnson and Mary E. Connors, *The Etiology and Treatment of Bulimia Nervosa: A Biopsychosocial Perspective* (New York: Basic Books, 1987), 149.

2. Some researchers divide women into those who feel pain during self-injury and those who do not, but they do not differentiate among types of self-injury. (See Mark J. Russ et al., "Pain Perception in Self-Injurious Patients with Borderline Personality Disorder," *Biological Psychiatry* 32 [1992]; and Mark J. Russ et al., "Subtypes of Self-Injurious Patients with Borderline Personality Disorder," *American Journal of Psychia-*

try 150, no. 12 [December 1993], 1869–1871.) I have not found such a division. Self-injury may or may not cause pain, depending on a woman's prior emotional state and on the type of self-injury she uses at a given time.

3. The statement concerning cutting is based on my own research as well as on conclusions drawn by Judith Himber in her 1993 dissertation "Blood Can Say Things: The Experience of Self-Cutting," Massachusetts School of Professional Psychology, 92; and by Armando R. Favazza in *Bodies Under Siege: Self-Mutilation and Body Modification in Culture and Psychiatry*, 2nd ed. (Baltimore: The Johns Hopkins University Press, 1996), 272–273. The statement concerning picking is drawn solely from my own research.

4. In "Female Habitual Self-Mutilators," *Acta Psychiatrica Scandinavia* 79 (1989), 286, A. R. Favazza and K. Conterio have written on cutting as associated with menstruation, starting only close to or after menarche. This does seem to be true of the women I interviewed. Studies of postmenopausal women who self-injure are needed to see if the observations of cutting subsiding around menopause are true for many women or only a few.

5. Mary V. Seeman, "Psychopathology in Women and Men: Focus on Female Hormones," *American Journal of Psychiatry* 154, no. 12 (December 1997), 1643–1644.

6. Ruta Mazelis, "SIV: Programs, Rituals, and Disbelief," in *The Cutting Edge: A Newsletter for Women Living with Self-Inflicted Violence*, vol. 8, no. 1 (29) (Spring 1997), 2.

7. Norman L. Faberow, "Indirect Self-Destructive Behavior: Classification and Characteristics," 19; and Robert E. Litman, "Psychodynamics of Indirect Self-Destructive Behavior," 32, in Norman L. Faberow, ed., *The Many Faces of Suicide: Indirect Self-Destructive Behavior* (New York: McGraw-Hill Book Company, 1980).

8. Penelope K. Trickett and Frank W. Putnam, "Impact of Child Sexual Abuse on Females: Toward a Developmental, Psychobiological Integration," *Psychological Science* 4, no. 2 (March 1993), 83.

9. Of course many, perhaps most, abusive relationships have nothing to do with self-injury by proxy, and even when they do, the abusive partner is responsible for his or her actions.

10. The idea that all sensations and some feelings, especially anger, are muted by layers of fat comes from the report of a woman cited in Jean M. Goodwin and Reina Attias, "Eating Disorders in Survivors of Multimodal Childhood Abuse," in Richard P. Kluft and Catherine G. Fine, eds., *Clinical Perspectives on Multiple Personality Disorder* (Washington, D.C.: American Psychiatric Press, 1993), 337. This woman's report corresponds with findings of muted activity in the autonomic nervous system associated with increased body fat. H. R. Peterson et al., "Body Fat and the Activity of the Autonomic Nervous System," *New England Journal of Medicine* 318 (1988), 1077–1083, as cited in Kluft and Fine, 337.

11. One study discusses women who, in order to continue injecting, substitute other drugs or tap water if their drug of choice is not available, or simply draw their own blood in and out of the needle. Some drug users call such women "needle freaks,"

recognizing that these women's need for needles is independent of their need for drugs. See David G. Levine, "'Needle Freaks': Compulsive Self-Injection by Drug Users," *American Journal of Psychiatry* 131, no. 3 (March 1974), 297.

12. Some of the functions were added by readers who critiqued chapter drafts, or were gleaned from David K. Sakheim and Lorraine Stanek, "Assessment of Self Injurious Coping Behaviors," in *Raising Issue*, special edition (Fall 1994), 1–15.

Chapter 2

1. Leon Eisenberg, "The Social Construction of the Human Brain," *American Journal of Psychiatry* 152, no. 11 (November 1995), 1563; E. R. Kandel and J. H. Schwartz, *Principles of Neural Science* (New York: Elsevier, 1985). Cited in Bessel A. van der Kolk and Onno van der Hart, "Pierre Janet and the Breakdown of Adaptation in Psychological Trauma," *American Journal of Psychiatry* 46, no. 12 (December 1989), 1534.

2. Michael A Schwartz et al., "Psychotic Experience and Disordered Thinking: A Reappraisal from New Perspectives," *The Journal of Nervous and Mental Disease* 185, no. 3 (1997), 183.

3. Michael D. De Bellis et al., "Developmental Traumatology: Biological Stress Systems and Brain Development in Maltreated Children with PTSD, Part II: The Relationship between Characteristics of Trauma and Psychiatric Symptoms and Adverse Brain Development in Maltreated Children and Adolescents with PTSD," *Biological Psychiatry*, 1999, in press; Murray B. Stein et al., "Neuroanatomical and Neuroendocrine Correlates in Adulthood of Severe Sexual Abuse in Childhood," *American College of Neuropsychopharmacology Abstracts* 33 (1994), 53, as discussed by Martin H. Teicher, "The Effects of Abuse on Brain Development," talk presented at the Academic Conference, McLean Hospital, Belmont, Massachusetts, January 24, 1997.

4. Stein, "Neuroanatomical and Neuroendocrine Correlates," as cited in Teicher, "The Effects of Abuse."

5. Personal communication with William A. Kadish, M.D., June, 1998.

6. See Bessel A. van der Kolk, *Psychological Trauma* (Washington, D.C.: American Psychiatric Press, 1987), 50–51.

7. Bessel A. van der Kolk et al., "Childhood Origins of Self-Destructive Behavior," *American Journal of Psychiatry* 148, no. 12 (December 1991), 1669; and Bessel A. van der Kolk and Rita E. Fisler, "Childhood Abuse and Neglect and Loss of Self-Regulation," *Bulletin of the Menninger Clinic* 58, no. 2 (1994), 151.

8. Bessel A. van der Kolk, *Psychological Trauma*, 68–69.

9. Michael D. de Bellis et al., "Urinary Catecholamine Excretion in Sexually Abused Girls," *Journal of the American Academy of Child and Adolescent Psychiatry* 33, no. 3 (March/April 1994), 324.

10. Michael D. de Bellis et al., "Hypothalamic-Pituitary-Adrenal Axis Dysregulation in Sexually Abused Girls," *Journal of Clinical Endocrinology and Metabolism* 78, no. 2 (1994), 249–255; Michael D. de Bellis et al., "Urinary Catecholamine Excretion in Sexually Abused Girls," 320–326; Heidi S. Resnick et al., "Effect of Previous Trauma on

Acute Plasma Cortisol Level Following Rape," *American Journal of Psychiatry* 152, no. 11 (November 1995), 1676; Daphne Simeon et al., "Self-Mutilation in Personality Disorders: Psychological and Biological Correlates," *American Journal of Psychiatry* 149, no. 2 (February 1992), 226; and Bessel A. van der Kolk et al., "Fluoxetine in Posttraumatic Stress Disorder," *Journal of Clinical Psychiatry* 55 (1994), 517–522.

11. Bessel A. van der Kolk et al., "Childhood Origins of Self-Destructive Behavior," 1665.

12. Bessel A. Van der Kolk, "The Body Keeps the Score: Memory and the Evolving Psychobiology of Posttraumatic Stress," *Harvard Review of Psychiatry* 1, no. 5 (1994), 253–265.

13. Bessel A. van der Kolk, "The Body Keeps the Score," 257.

14. This is Barbara's experience and is only one of many possible physical sensations resulting from prior abuse. Informally, mental-health professionals often call such sensations "body memories," although some sensations resulting from prior trauma are officially classified as "conversion disorder" or "somatization disorder." See the Diagnostic and Statistical Manual of Mental Disorders (DSM-IV), 4th ed. (Washington, D.C.: American Psychiatric Association, 1994), 452–457 and 446–450 respectively.

15. Bessel A. van der Kolk, "The Trauma Spectrum: The Interaction of Biological and Social Events in the Genesis of the Trauma Response," *Journal of Traumatic Stress* 1, no. 3 (1988), 278.

16. Bessel A. van der Kolk, *Psychological Trauma*, 72.

17. Bessel A. van der Kolk, "The Trauma Spectrum," 273–290.

18. Bessel A. van der Kolk, "The Trauma Spectrum," 278 and 285–286.

19. Bessel A. Van der Kolk and Jose Saporta, "The Biological Response to Psychic Trauma: Mechanisms and Treatment of Intrusion and Numbing," *Anxiety Research* 4 (1991), 207.

20. Bessel A. van der Kolk, "The Trauma Spectrum," 285–286.

21. Bessel A. van der Kolk and Rita E. Fisler, "Childhood Abuse and Neglect and Loss of Self-Regulation," *Bulletin of the Menninger Clinic* 58, no. 2 (1994), 146.

22. The intensity of the central nervous system's response to the trauma predicts the long-term outcome. See Bessel A. van der Kolk, "The Trauma Spectrum: The Interaction of Biological and Social Events in the Genesis of the Trauma Response," 274.

23. Physical arousal is an automatic response unrelated, in women, to whether they want sex or not, and a woman can become physiologically aroused without wanting sex. Lubrication helps prevent worse physical damage during rape. Yet, women often feel guilty if they become lubricated during a rape, thinking that this is a sign of having "wanted" sex and that this sign encouraged the rapist. Arousal of any kind may add to young girls' feelings of guilt.

24. James A. Chu, "The Therapeutic Roller Coaster: Dilemmas in the Treatment of Childhood Abuse Survivors," *Journal of Psychotherapy Practice and Research* 1, no. 4 (Fall 1992), 354; and Bessel A. van der Kolk et al., "Childhood Origins of Self-Destructive Behavior," *American Journal of Psychiatry* 148, no. 12 (December 1991), 1667.

25. Bessel A. van der Kolk and Rita E. Fisler, "Childhood Abuse and Neglect and Loss of Self-Regulation," 157.

26. Judith Himber, "Blood Can Say Things: The Experience of Self-Cutting," dissertation, Massachusetts School of Professional Psychology, 1993, 112.

27. Judith Himber, "Blood Can Say Things: The Experience of Self-Cutting," 118.

28. Barent W. Walsh and Paul M. Rosen, *Self-Mutilation: Theory, Research, and Treatment* (New York: The Guilford Press, 1988), 65.

29. *Webster's New Collegiate Dictionary* (Springfield, Mass.: G. & C. Merriam Company, 1979).

30. Suggested by Janice McLane's article, "The Voice on the Skin: Self-Mutilation and Merleau-Ponty's Theory of Language," *Hypatia* 11, no. 4 (Fall 1996), 110.

31. Elaine (Hilberman) Carmen et al., "Victims of Violence and Psychiatric Illness," *American Journal of Psychiatry* 141, no. 3 (March 1984), 380; Lenore C. Terr, "Childhood Traumas: An Outline and Overview," *American Journal of Psychiatry* 148, no. 1 (January 1991), 17.

32. Elaine (Hilberman) Carmen et al., "Victims of Violence and Psychiatric Illness," 382; V. E. Pollock et al., "Childhood Antecedents of Antisocial Behavior: Parental Alcoholism and Physical Abusiveness," *American Journal of Psychiatry* 147, no. 10 (October 1990), 1292.

33. Robin Connors, "Self-Injury in Trauma Survivors: 1. Functions and Meanings," *American Journal of Orthopsychiatry* 66, no. 2 (April 1996), 202.

34. Bessel A. van der Kolk, "Childhood Abuse and Neglect and Loss of Self-Regulation," 145. Presentation at the 15th Annual Menninger Winter Psychiatry Conference, March 7–22, 1993, Park City, Utah.

35. A. J. Reiss and J. A. Roth, "Patterns of Violence in American Society," in A. J. Reiss and J. A. Roth, eds., *Understanding and Preventing Violence* (Washington, D.C.: National Academy Press, 1993), 42–97, as cited in Peter M. Marzuk, "Violence, Crime and Mental Illness: How Strong a Link?" *Archives of General Psychiatry* 53 (June 1996), 482.

36. Cathy Spatz Widom, "The Cycle of Violence," *Science* 244 (April 1989), 160–162.

37. S. Yochelson and S. Samenow, *The Criminal Personality* (New York: Aronson, 1976), as cited in Joel Paris, "Antisocial and Borderline Personality Disorders: Two Separate Diagnoses or Two Aspects of the Same Psychopathology?" *Comprehensive Psychiatry* 38, no. 4 (July/August 1997), 237; G. E. Vaillant, "Sociopathy as a Human Process," *Archives of General Psychiatry* 32, (1975), 178–183. Incarceration itself can lead to responses similar to those accompanying childhood abuse: entrapment followed by helplessness, hopelessness, and explosive anger and frustration with no permissible outlet for these emotions.

38. P. F. Brain and M. Haug, "Hormonal and Neurochemical Correlates of Various Forms of Animal 'Aggression,'" *Psychoneuroendocrinology* 17, no. 6 (1993), 538–539; and David R. Rubinow and Peter J. Schmidt, "Androgens, Brain, and Behavior," *American Journal of Psychiatry* 153, no. 8 (August 1996), 980–981.

Chapter 4

1. Feeling like two people can also be based on experiences with alter identities. Some self-injuring women who have alter identities arrange that an alter identity go to work on a regular basis, or feel that a different part of them is the worker. Because "someone else" goes to work, some women are able to build a well-defined wall between work and all other aspects of their lives. Going to work then becomes a way of blocking everything else out and entering a life separate from any reminder of another, troubled life.

2. Observation made by Dawn Balcazar, Ph.D., psychologist at the Trauma Center, Human Resource Institute, Brookline, Massachusetts.

3. Nine women said that no one knows, one was unsure how much her colleagues knew, three said that some knew, and two had each told one selected colleague.

4. Three women who had never told anyone at the workplace reacted dispassionately to the question, "What do you think might happen if you told an employer or colleague?" These women spoke mainly about their employers, saying that their employers would not want to know about self-injury or simply that it would be inappropriate to tell an employer. In two cases, employers had already indicated that they did not want to know any details about why the women had been hospitalized.

5. Seven women revealed that work affected self-injury, two said that self-injury affects productivity, and six said that neither was the case.

6. Of the nine women who self-injure at work, the five who do not self-injure as a result of work also do not refer to their work as highly stressful. The four who self-injure in response to work situations all refer to their work as highly stressful.

7. Karen Conterio, personal communication, October, 1995.

8. Examples include Dusty Miller, psychologist and author of *Women Who Hurt Themselves: A Book of Hope and Understanding*; Robin Connors, counselor and author (with Kristy Trautmann) of *Understanding Self-Injury: A Workbook for Adults*; and Annie G. Rogers, psychologist and author of *A Shining Affliction: A Story of Harm and Healing in Psychotherapy*.

9. "Employers will need to provide 'reasonable accommodation' to individuals with disabilities. This includes steps such as job restructuring and modification of equipment," cited from the *Americans with Disabilities Act Requirements Fact Sheet*, U.S. Department of Justice, Civil Rights Division (Washington, D.C.: U.S. Government Printing Office).

Chapter 5

1. This conforms with other research showing that "sexual problems" are a significant aftermath of childhood sexual abuse. See Diana M. Elliott and John Briere, "Sexual Abuse Trauma among Professional Women: Validating the Trauma Symptom Checklist-40 (TSC-40)," *Child Abuse and Neglect* 16 (1992), 396.

2. Self-injury or scars are or were sources of strife in the relationships of all but four of my informants who currently have or have ever had steady partners. Of those four — two heterosexual and two lesbian — two were not injuring themselves during the years of the relationship.

3. Judith L. Herman, "Considering Sex Offenders: A Model of Addiction," *Signs: Journal of Women in Culture and Society* 13 (1988), 695–724, as cited in Judith L. Herman, "Sequelae of Prolonged and Repeated Trauma: Evidence for a Complex Posttraumatic Syndrome (DESNOS)," in Jonathan R. T. Davidson and Edna B. Foa, eds., *Posttraumatic Stress Disorder: DSM-IV and Beyond* (Washington, D.C.: American Psychiatric Press, 1993), 223.

4. J. Kaufman and E. Zigler, "Do Abused Children Become Abusive Parents?" *American Journal of Orthopsychiatry* 57 (1987), 186–192, as cited in Judith L. Herman, "Sequelae of Prolonged and Repeated Trauma: Evidence for a Complex Posttraumatic Syndrome (DESNOS)," 223.

5. Bryon Egeland et al., "Breaking the Cycle of Abuse," *Child Development* 59 (1988), 1080–1088, a study of 161 mothers, 47 of whom were physically abused as children and 114 of whom were not.

Chapter 7

1. Iris Weaver, who formerly self-injured and is the author of a newsletter for abused women (*Roots of Healing*, P.O. Box 2441, Quincy, MA 02269-2441); women who responded to questions on the internet site http://palace.net/-llama/selfinjury; and women who contributed to *Self-Harm: Perspectives from Personal Experience* (October 1994), Louise Roxanne Pembroke, ed., published by Survivors Speak Out, 34 Osnaburgh Street, London NW1 3ND, England.

2. Suggestion made by Deb Martinson, who provides the tokens.

3. Ruta Mazelis, "SIV: Expanding Our Options," in *The Cutting Edge: A Newsletter for Women Living with Self-Inflicted Violence* 7, no. 1 (25), (Spring 1996), 3.

4. Deb Martinson, paraprofessional counselor and provider of web site information on self-injury, drawing on her experience with DBT as a client, and the experiences of other DBT participants.

5. For example, see Hani Raoul Khouzam and Nancy Jane Donnelly, "Remission of Self-Mutilation in a Patient with Borderline Personality during Resperidone Therapy," *Journal of Nervous and Mental Disease* 185, no. 5 (May 1997), 348–349.

6. See Armando R. Favazza, *Bodies Under Siege: Self-Mutilation and Body Modification in Culture and Psychiatry,* 2nd ed., (Baltimore: The Johns Hopkins University Press, 1996), 290–291.

7. Annie G. Rogers, "Writing on their Bodies I: Understanding Self-Mutilation with Adolescent Girls through Creative Writing in Psychotherapy," paper presented at Harvard Medical School Conference, "Child and Adolescent Self-Destruction," Boston, Mass., February 3, 1996, and at Trinity College: Psychology and Women's Studies Departments, Dublin, Ireland, April 25, 1996.

8. Roger K. Pitman et al., "Emotional Processing during Eye Movement Desensitization and Reprocessing Therapy of Vietnam Veterans with Chronic Posttraumatic Stress Disorder," *Comprehensive Psychiatry* 37, no. 6 (November/December) 1996, 419–429.

9. Malcolm J. Macculloch and Philip Feldman cite eight controlled trials in "Eye Movement Desensitisation Treatment Utilises the Positive Visceral Element of the Investigatory Reflex to Inhibit the Memories of Post-Traumatic Stress Disorder: a Theoretical Analysis," *British Journal of Psychiatry* 169 (1996), 571–572.

10. Margaret M. Scheck et al., "Brief Psychological Intervention with Traumatized Young Women: The Efficacy of Eye Movement Desensitization and Reprocessing," *Journal of Traumatic Stress* 11, no. 1 (1998), 25–41.

11. Sandra A. Wilson et al., "Eye Movement Desensitization and Reprocessing (EMDR) Treatment for Psychologically Traumatized Individuals," *Journal of Consulting and Clinical Psychology*, 63, no. 6 (1995), 935.

12. Personal communications with Patti Levin, LICSW, Psy.D., May 27, 1998, and Deborah L. Korn, Psy.D., July 20, 1998.

13. Information on these therapies stem from Mary Sykes Wylie, "Going for the Cure," *The Family Therapy Networker* (July/August 1996), 26–29.

14. *Diagnostic and Statistical Manual of Mental Disorders*, 4th ed., (Washington, D.C.: American Psychiatric Association, 1994), 654.

15. The suggestions in this paragraph stem from Robin Connors, "Self-Injury in Trauma Survivors: 2. Levels of Clinical Response," *American Journal of Orthopsychiatry* 66 (2), (April 1996), 209 and 211. In a 1998 conference on self-injury in women and girls sponsored by the Center for Mental Health Services, two related recommendations were made: 1. Therapists and clients should be partners in healing; and 2. A minimum of 33 percent of people involved in large-scale treatment planning for self-injury (program design, evaluation, and administration) should be current or former clients.

Epilogue

1. See Fakir Musafar, "Body Play: State of Grace or Sickness?" in Armando R. Favazza, *Bodies Under Siege: Self-Mutilation and Body Modification in Culture and Psychiatry*, 2nd ed. (Baltimore: The Johns Hopkins University Press, 1996), 329; and interview with Raelyn Gallina in V. Vale and Andrea Juno, eds., *Modern Primitives: An Investigation of Contemporary Adornment and Ritual* (San Francisco: Re/Search Publications, 1989), 105.

2. Interview with Genesis and Paula P-Orridge in V. Vale and Andrea Juno, eds., *Modern Primitives*, 164.

3. From interview as above with Genesis P-Orridge in V. Vale and Andrea Juno, eds., *Modern Primitives*, 164.

4. Interview with Fakir Musafar in V. Vale and Andrea Juno, eds., *Modern Primitives*, 6–7.

5. Fakir Musafar, ed., *Body Play: The Self-Images of Fakir Musafar, 1950–1980* (San Francisco, Calif.: Limited edition published privately by Insight Books, 1982), unpaginated.

6. V. Vale and Andrea Juno, eds., *Modern Primitives*, 35.

7. Giles Constable, *Attitudes toward Self-Inflicted Suffering in the Middle Ages* (Brookline, Mass.: Hellenic College Press, 1982), 7–8.

8. Rosemary Curb and Nancy Manahen, eds., *Lesbian Nuns: Breaking Silence* (n.p.: The Naiad Press, Inc., 1985), 213.

9. Constable, *Attitudes toward Self-Inflicted Suffering in the Middle Ages*, 12.

10. Constable, *Attitudes toward Self-Inflicted Suffering in the Middle Ages*, 15.

11. Constable, *Attitudes toward Self-Inflicted Suffering in the Middle Ages*, 15.

12. Constable, *Attitudes toward Self-Inflicted Suffering in the Middle Ages*, 15.

13. From a translation of the first of Saint Veronica's five autobiographies and cited in Rudolph M. Bell, *Holy Anorexia* (Chicago: University of Chicago Press, 1985), 60.

14. Rudolph M. Bell, *Holy Anorexia*, 61, citing from Saint Veronica's second autobiography.

15. Rudolph M. Bell, *Holy Anorexia*, 73, citing from a five-volume edition of Sister Veronica's writings published 1969–1974.

16. This information stems from an account undated (but written between 1947 and 1958) of the saint's life by E. J. Dingwall called "St. Mary Magdalene de'Pazzi: She Who Got Slapped," in *Very Peculiar People: Portrait Studies in the Queer, the Abnormal and the Uncanny*, London: Rider and Company, 144. Dingwall's chapter is based on seventeenth- and nineteenth-century sources.

17. Interview with Anton Lavey, *Modern Primitives*, 94.

18. Armando R. Favazza, *Bodies Under Siege*, 2nd ed., 26–28.

19. The *New Catholic Encyclopedia* [n.v.], 145, as cited in Robert Robertson Ross and Hugh Bryan McKay, *Self-Mutilation* (Lexington, Mass.: D.C. Heath & Co., 1979), 46.

Index